Epilepsy Questions and Answers

*Written and edited by Professor Neil Buchanan
in conjunction with the New Zealand Epilepsy Association
and the Epilepsy Association of Tasmania*

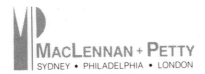
MacLennan + Petty
SYDNEY • PHILADELPHIA • LONDON

First published 1989

MacLennan & Petty Pty Limited
80 Reserve Road, Artarmon NSW 2064

© 1989 MacLennan & Petty Pty Limited

National library of Australia
Cataloguing-in-Publication data:

Buchanan, Neil, 1943−
Epilepsy questions & answers.
Includes index.

ISBN 0 86433 063 4.

1. Epilepsy − Popular works.   2. Epilepsy − Miscellanea.
I. Title.

616.8′53

Printed and bound in Australia

Contents

Introduction

This book is based upon questions asked of the field officers of the epilepsy associations in New Zealand and Tasmania. The text and the answers were prepared by Neil Buchanan in association with Deborah Marsh (New Zealand) and Colleen Martin (Tasmania). We are indebted to Drs Peter Procopis and Ernest Somerville for their comments and advice on the text and to Robyn Kenna for typing (many times) the manuscript.

It is hoped that this book will provide useful, practical information for people with epilepsy, their relatives, school teachers and health professionals. Naturally it does not provide answers to all possible questions, but serves as an introduction to the subject to be read in conjunction with other literature on epilepsy (see Appendix 1, Page 105).

Readers who have other questions which they feel could usefully be included in a book of this nature are invited to send them to Professor Buchanan, Westmead Hospital, Westmead, Sydney 2145, Australia. This might allow a further edition to be produced in due course.

Royalties from the sales of this book go directly to the New Zealand Epilepsy Association and the Epilepsy Association of Tasmania.

Professor Neil Buchanan
October 1988.

Chapter 1
What is Epilepsy?

An epileptic fit is due to an abnormal discharge of electrical activity produced by the nerve cells in the brain. This in turn produces an abnormal movement, sensation or thought process which is apparent to the person with epilepsy or an onlooker, and sometimes to both.

People with epilepsy lose control of their body, usually with complete or partial loss of consciousness, at various unexpected times. In other words, they may make movements without consciously wishing to do so and often without being aware of what is happening. The loss of conscious control may be referred to as an 'absence', 'blackout', 'convulsion', 'turn', 'seizure' or 'fit'. The most commonly used terms are seizure, convulsion and fit. All these terms mean the same thing, although seizure is currently the preferred term.

The frequency of fits reflects the severity of the epilepsy. Seizures differ from person to person: they range from being almost unnoticeable with the patient being 'absent' (in a trance and not 'with it') for a few seconds to seizures where the person may fall to the ground and jerk the arms and legs. Some people have frequent seizures and need to take medication regularly, while others may have only two or three convulsions in their whole lives.

About 80% of epilepsy will begin before the age of 20 years, and approximately 5% of children will have a fit at some time or other during childhood. The majority of these fits are related to fever (febrile convulsions) and are not associated with epilepsy as such. It is important to remember that a single fit does not imply a diagnosis of epilepsy – **by definition, epilepsy implies a tendency to recurrent seizures**.

Sadly, the diagnosis of epilepsy is often associated by patients and parents with a feeling that 'the end of the world' is at hand. This is not the case. Most people with epilepsy lead normal, productive lives. Even in the more serious types of epilepsy a great deal can be done to limit the consequences. Epilepsy in itself does not cause a person to be backward; persons with epilepsy are as intelligent as other people, although a small number may have some degree of brain damage which causes mental retardation as well as the fits. There may be some children who have learning problems and sometimes the medications used to treat epilepsy (anticonvulsants) may be sedating.

How many people have epilepsy?

Whilst this may seem a quite simple question, the answer is in fact uncertain. Because epilepsy is often a hidden condition which people are reticent to declare and as the diagnosis of epilepsy is not always clear, the frequency of the condition is probably underestimated. It is probable that in most Western societies epilepsy affects 1 out of every 100 people (1% of the population). This in fact makes epilepsy a quite common condition.

Does everyone who has a fit have epilepsy?

No. A fit (seizure, convulsion) is the main symptom of epilepsy. By definition, epilepsy implies having recurrent (more than one) seizures. Many people will have a single (isolated) seizure and not go on to develop epilepsy. Although it is known that some people who have had an isolated seizure will have further seizures and thus develop epilepsy, this occurs in the minority of such people. Probably about 5% of the population will have had isolated seizures (including febrile convulsions) as opposed to the 1% of the population who have epilepsy.

One of the worst things about my epilepsy is that I cannot get an explanation of what it is.

Many people with epilepsy find this frustrating. There is a lot of research yet to be done to explain exactly what goes on in the brain to cause epileptic seizures. As you will appreciate, it is very difficult to study the brain, except by indirect methods, as it is so well protected within the skull. This means that epilepsy research is a deal slower than any of us would like.

For those people in whom there is not an identifiable cause for their epilepsy, in other words where the cause is unknown (idiopathic epilepsy), it is believed that there is a chemical abnormality in the brain. It is felt, albeit not absolutely proven, that this is the cause of their epilepsy. One hopes that the chemical abnormality or abnormalities will be better understood in years to come.

Until this is understood and can be intelligibly explained to people with epilepsy, the frustration associated with the question 'What is epilepsy?' will persist.

There still seems to be an association in the minds of some people between epilepsy and madness. Is there any truth in this?

No there is not. Whilst there may be the occasional person with epilepsy who in addition has a psychiatric problem, this is extremely uncommon. There is no relationship between epilepsy and psychiatric illness.

People with epilepsy may have their fair share of psychological and psychosocial problems, but not frank psychiatric illness. In fact it has been shown that 'average' adults with epilepsy have a higher incidence of psychological problems than people without epilepsy or people with other neurological conditions. This may in part be due to community stigma and attitudes towards those with epilepsy.

Chapter 2
What are the Causes of Epilepsy?

There are many causes of epilepsy, which may vary with the age at which the seizures begin. As a generalization, it can be said that an epileptic fit occurs when, due to a sudden unusual release of energy (electrical activity) in the brain, its normal working is disturbed. The brain then fairly rapidly corrects itself and everything soon returns to normal.

From an explanatory point of view, although it may not be strictly medically acceptable, it is useful to divide epilepsy into two types: 1. primary epilepsy – idiopathic epilepsy; and 2. secondary epilepsy.

Primary epilepsy

The seizures in primary epilepsy may be identical to those in secondary epilepsy, but on examination of the brain with today's techniques, unlike secondary epilepsy, it is not possible to find an abnormality of brain tissue.

For many years this type of epilepsy has been called idiopathic epilepsy, which means that the cause is not understood. There are those who do not like the term 'idiopathic' epilepsy, as they argue that there must be a cause; it is just that we don't know what it is at present. It is probable that in idiopathic epilepsy there are abnormalities of chemicals in the cells of the area of brain tissue which is electrically abnormal. These chemical abnormalities are such that from time to time epileptic discharges may be produced. The exact nature of this chemical abnormality has yet to be understood.

Understanding this chemical abnormality is very important for two reasons:

- Firstly, it will provide a much better understanding of the nature of epilepsy.
- Secondly, it may allow the production of drugs (anticonvul-

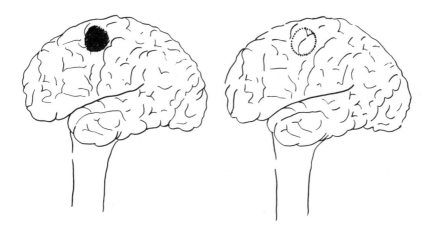

Figure 1. *The brain on the left has a clearly visible abnormality (secondary epilepsy) while the one on the right has an 'invisible' abnormality (primary, idiopathic epilepsy).*

sants, anti-epileptic drugs) specifically aimed at correcting the chemical abnormality.

Secondary epilepsy

Secondary epilepsy is an easier concept to grasp. It means that the symptoms, namely the fits, are secondary, or subsequent to, some obvious abnormality of the brain (see fig. 1). In other words, if you could look at the brain itself and examine it, either during life using x-ray techniques like CT or MRI scanning (see Chapter 4), or at autopsy, it would be possible to find an actual abnormality in the brain. The person may have been born with this abnormality of the brain or it may be a scar related to brain damage at birth, a head injury and so on.

It can be fairly easily understood that if there is a structural abnormality of brain tissue, then the brain cells surrounding that abnormality will be somewhat misshapen and possibly functioning abnormally as a result. If you have a scar somewhere on your body, glance at it and notice how it pulls the surrounding skin and tissues in various directions.

Some of the particular causes of epilepsy include:

- Anoxia (hypoxia), i.e. lack of oxygen to the brain.
- Brain damage.
- Brain tumours.
- Previous brain infections.

Is epilepsy inherited?

It is unwise to talk about 'epilepsy' as such. There are many different types of epilepsy; some are inherited and the majority are not. For example, someone who has epilepsy as a result of a head injury, meningitis or a brain operation quite obviously does not have epilepsy in their genetic make-up and cannot pass it on to their children.

As a generalization it can be said that if one parent has epilepsy, the chances of one of the children having epilepsy are no greater than in the population at large (i.e. 1%). If both parents have epilepsy, the chance of a child having it are about 10 per cent. If the epilepsy in the parent(s) is due to a head injury, meningitis, birth trauma etc., it is not handed on to their children.

In childhood absence epilepsy (petit mal) about one-third of patients have a family history of either childhood absence epilepsy or tonic–clonic seizures (grand mal). In identical twins for example, if one twin has childhood absences there is a 75% chance that the other twin will also be affected and 85% of other twins will show the EEG features of this type of epilepsy. In photosensitive epilepsy, about 25% of siblings of people with this form of epilepsy show EEG changes of photosensitivity. There are also a number of rare conditions which cause epilepsy which may be inherited.

Are febrile convulsions related to epilepsy?

With the exception of rare instances of severe and prolonged febrile convulsions, which may last for several hours, simple febrile convulsions do not lead to epilepsy.

Febrile convulsions can be divided into so-called simple and complex febrile convulsions. Simple febrile convulsions last less than 15 minutes and are usually tonic–clonic (grand mal) seizures. Complex febrile convulsions usually last more than 15 minutes and may affect only one side of the body. Children who have complex febrile convulsions may be developmentally delayed or have some evidence of a neurological problem. Both these features, in their own right, are associated with a higher incidence of epilepsy. Thus it is not surprising that those who have had complex febrile convulsions may subsequently develop epilepsy.

It is important for the parents of epileptic children to be aware that fever is a provoking factor for seizures. This means that young children, who normally have a lot of infections in the first 5 or 6 years of life, may show a deterioration in seizure control when they have an infection and a fever. For some children this does not present a problem but for others there may be a flurry of fits lasting for a few days whilst the youngster is unwell. The first time that this occurs, parents think that they have lost control of the child's epilepsy and often become very anxious. This is best dealt with by explanation, aided by the liberal use of paracetamol to bring the fever down. Recurrent seizure exacerbations with fever may need to be dealt with by using rectal diazepam (Valium) either to prevent the seizures or when the first seizure has occurred.

Can you bring on a fit?

Yes you can. There are probably three types of fits that can be 'brought on'. The first are seizures which are related to stress (see page 81); these may occur when a person is in a stressful situation or is anticipating such a situation.

The second type of seizure is called a pseudoseizure (false fit). These usually occur in people who have epilepsy although they may occur in people who do not, but who have witnessed seizures. Pseudoseizures are 'brought on' subconsciously and are attention seeking in nature. There is always a reason for someone behaving in this way, although the cause may take some long time to discover. Pseudoseizures are sometimes rather bizarre and fairly obvious to the experienced observer, but usually they are fairly similar to the person's regular seizures. This makes the diagnosis much less obvious and for that reason pseudoseizures should always be thought of in patients in whom seizures get inexorably worse, usually in the face of more and more medication. If the diagnosis cannot be made by simple observation, video-telemetry is needed so that the seizure can be observed on video and recorded on the EEG at the same time. If the EEG is quite normal during the suspected seizure, it is quite likely that it is a pseudoseizure. Management consists of finding the psychological reason for this sort of behaviour and trying to deal with it whilst reducing anticonvulsant medication to a bare minimum.

The third type of seizure occurs in children with photosensitive epilepsy who may occasionally bring on fits by purposely sitting very close to the TV or by waving their hands in front of their faces, to produce alternating light and shade, thus producing a seizure.

Since taking the contraceptive pill and therefore no longer ovulating, I have had far fewer complex partial seizures. Is ovulating the reason I had seizures?

It is unlikely that ovulating as such is the cause of the seizures. On the other hand, in your case, the hormonal changes associated with ovulation may make your seizures worse. To confuse the issue further, there are some people in whom the oral contraceptive pill appears to make seizures worse.

The whole relationship between seizures and hormonal balance is poorly understood. Moreover, it is very difficult to study as there is not necessarily a good relationship between the blood levels of various hormones and their effects in the tissues, especially the brain.

From a practical point of view, if your seizures are improved with the oral contraceptive pill that's fine. However, if the reverse had occurred, you would have needed to find an alternative form of contraception.

If I am photosensitive to TV, will I also be sensitive to changes in light and strobe lights?

Yes it is possible, although TV is by far the commonest photosensitive (light) provoking factor. Bright sunlight, light reflected off water, strobe lights, alternating light and shade and computer games may all be provoking factors in the photosensitive individual. Video display units are not a problem in this regard.

My son had his first seizure at fourteen. What chances are there of him having another one? His first seizure was after a long trip on which he suffered travel and sea sickness. Could this seizure have been caused by that or do you think he will get epilepsy?

Firstly a single seizure does not constitute epilepsy, so your son does not have epilepsy. Secondly, isolated seizures such as your son had, may or may not be associated with a provoking factor.

When associated with a provoking factor, of which severe fatigue is one (see page 81), the chances of an unprovoked seizure recurrence are slight. However, if the person is again subject to the same provocation, a seizure may recur.

We all have the potential to have seizures if sufficiently provoked. If one's seizure threshold is lowered sufficiently, a seizure may ensue. The provoking factors discussed on pages 81−2 all serve to lower the seizure threshold and thus predispose to seizures.

Does puberty increase the incidence of seizures in any way?

Perhaps surprisingly there is no clear-cut answer to this commonly asked question. The reason that the question is so often posed is that it is generally believed that there is a relationship between the two. Despite this there is no proof of such a relationship. From a practical point of view, it may well be that for some girls there is a deterioration in seizure control associated with the onset of puberty. This does not seem to occur in boys. When a deterioration in seizure control, assumed to be associated with puberty, occurs it is not usually responsive to increased anticonvulsant therapy. The deterioration usually lasts months to a year.

My son had a seizure after his second whooping cough (pertussis) injection. He now has established epilepsy. Was the vaccination the cause?

Whooping cough itself, especially if severe, may cause some brain damage. This occurs very rarely in this day and age, thanks largely to a successful vaccination programme. None of today's parents of young children and many doctors presently in practice, will have seen the devastating effects of whooping cough.

A number of studies have looked at the relationship between whooping cough vaccination and subsequent epilepsy. There does appear to be a relationship in a very small number of children. Despite this, whooping cough vaccination is still strongly recommended as severe whooping cough is such an unpleasant and dangerous illness.

Having said this, if a child has a severe reaction to their first dose of pertussis vaccine, especially a seizure, further doses should not be given. Pertussis vaccine is being further purified and the incidence of vaccine reactions can be expected to fall.

My 15-year-old daughter has had epilepsy for 8 months. I have a friend who has a brain tumour and I am worried that my daughter has the same thing.

Even if you did not have a friend with a brain tumour, you might still worry about this possible association.

Brain tumours are an uncommon cause of epilepsy in all age groups, but especially in children. Signs of a tumour are likely to be found on clinical examination but it may be necessary to do a CT scan (see page 24) to exclude this.

My son has had epilepsy for 4 years. I can accept that. But I feel guilty that it may be due to one of a number of bangs to his head which occurred in early childhood.

There can be very few children who do not have a few bangs to the head in early childhood. If such bangs caused epilepsy, then most children would have epilepsy as opposed to the 1% who have the condition. Head injuries certainly can lead to subsequent epilepsy, but need to be severe and associated with prolonged loss of consciousness.

Is there a relationship between epilepsy and allergy?

No there is not.

Chapter 3

What Types of Seizures are There?

The classification of epilepsy has become quite complicated with a number of suggested classifications over the past two decades. **There is now a general feeling that it is better to think in terms of the epilepsies or epilepsy syndromes, rather than of epilepsy** *per se.* Although there is not a universally accepted classification of the epilepsies, especially in childhood, there is general agreement that many are distinctive, not only in terms of their symptoms and management, but also with regard to outlook.

Thus, at present, epilepsy can be discussed in two ways:

1. By discussing **seizure type**. In other words, a person may have tonic–clonic (grand mal) seizures. This, however, does not define precisely the sort of epilepsy that they have, as tonic–clonic seizures may occur in more than one type of epilepsy.
2. By discussing the **type of epilepsy, or the epilepsy syndrome**, which that person has. Thus a child may have infantile spasms as the type of epilepsy, but exhibit myoclonic jerks and tonic–clonic seizures as their seizure type.

This chapter discusses the various types of seizures which can occur and the various epilepsy syndromes are shown in table 1.

From a practical point of view, seizures can be divided into generalized and partial seizures. A **generalized seizure** implies that abnormal electrical activity involves both halves of the brain (cerebral hemispheres) from the outset.

On the other hand, **partial seizures** start in one cerebral hemisphere and the electrical activity remains in that area, not spreading to the other side of the brain. Thus the term 'partial seizure' means that only part of the brain is involved.

As a working rule, a generalized seizure which involves the whole brain is associated with losing consciousness. In partial seizures, consciousness is retained to a greater or lesser extent. In some partial seizures, consciousness may be retained initially but

Epileptic syndromes in newborn babies

Benign neonatal convulsions
Early myoclonic encephalopathy
Other epileptic syndromes in newborn babies

Epileptic syndromes in infancy* and childhood

Infantile spasms
Benign myoclonic epilepsy in infants
Severe myoclonic epilepsy in infants
Myoclonic epilepsy in non-progressive encephalopathies
Epileptic seizures in children with inborn errors of metabolism
Myoclonic – astatic epilepsy of early childhood
The Lennox-Gastaut syndrome

Epileptic syndromes in childhood

Childhood absence epilepsy
Epilepsy with myoclonic absences
Epilepsy with generalized convulsive seizures
Benign partial epilepsies of childhood
Benign partial epilepsy with centro-temporal spikes
Benign epilepsy of childhood with occipital spikes
Benign psychomotor epilepsy
The Landau–Kleffner syndrome
Epilepsy with continuous spikes and waves during slow sleep

Epileptic syndromes in childhood and adolescence

Photosensitive epilepsies
Juvenile absence epilepsy
Juvenile myoclonic epilepsy
Epilepsy with grand mal on awakening
Benign partial seizures of adolescence
Progressive myoclonic epilepsy in childhood and adolescence

* Infancy implies that period from 1 to 12 months of life.

Table 1. *A summary of the epilepsy syndromes in childhood and adolescence. This exemplifies firstly that there are many different types of epilepsy and secondly that they are, at least in part, age related. Just looking at a list like this should discourage people from talking about 'epilepsy' as an all-encompassing condition.*

then the fit may become secondarily generalized and the patient will become unconscious in association with a major generalized fit.

There are a number of different types of seizures (fits) which will be discussed in some detail. However, before doing so, a general comment is warranted. **It is of considerable importance that people with epilepsy should know precisely what type of seizures and what type of epilepsy they have.** It is not good enough to say 'I have epilepsy'. You should be able to say, 'I have complex partial seizures (temporal lobe epilepsy)' or 'my child has infantile spasms'. The reason that you as an epileptic, or the parent of an epileptic child, should know this is that the outlook for the various types of epilepsy differs. Equally important, **from a public relations point of view, people with epilepsy or parents of epileptic children need to be advocates for epilepsy**. As we have already discussed, the general public is ill-informed about epilepsy. They believe all epilepsy is a tonic–clonic fit as they have seen on television. Only by being precise about **your** epilepsy will you be able to educate those around you about epilepsy and its implications.

Tonic–clonic seizures (Grand mal seizures; major generalized seizures)

Grand mal (tonic–clonic) seizures are the commonest type of seizure. About 70% to 80% of children with epilepsy have grand mal fits. A tonic–clonic fit may begin without warning or may be preceded by an aura.

An **aura** is a sensation which precedes loss of consciousness and is actually the beginning of the fit. This may be a regular event for some people, but not for others. The nature of the aura will depend on the area of the brain in which the fit begins. Some people may exhibit unusual behaviour or be somewhat out of sorts before an attack.

At the start of the fit there is a sudden loss of consciousness. If at that time the patient is standing, he or she will fall to the ground. This is quickly followed by generalized rigidity (stiffening) of the body, called the **tonic phase** of the fit. This is then followed by a generalized jerking of the body, the **clonic phase**. During the clonic phase patients may bite their tongue, pass urine or pass a motion. These three events occur less often in children than in adults.

During the tonic phase, when the body is rigid, the face and lips may go blue (cyanosis) as the patient is unable to breathe because of the stiffening of the body. Thereafter, breathing becomes jerky during the clonic phase and the cyanosis (blueness) lessens. The clonic movements then gradually settle down and the patient becomes relaxed and limp. After a tonic–clonic fit the patient may recover rapidly, but if it has been a long fit, they may go into a deep sleep. Associated with recovery there may be feelings of weakness, headache or fatigue and some people may be confused and irritable. In addition, some people may injure themselves during a fit.

When a number of grand mal convulsions follow each other in rapid succession, the situation becomes serious and is called **status epilepticus**. This implies that the epilepsy is continuous and will not stop spontaneously. This is a medical emergency and will be discussed later in this chapter.

Absences (petit mal seizures)

For years the term petit mal has been used to describe this form of seizure. This is no longer recommended and the term absences is preferred. The reason for this is that the term petit mal is often used incorrectly by patients to describe a whole miscellany of fits that are not grand mal, but nor are they absences. It is therefore a confusing term.

Absences are a form of generalized epilepsy. In a petit mal absence, there is either a decrease or suppression in mental function which begins and ends abruptly. Attacks may last for 5 to 30 seconds and occasionally longer. They often occur many times a day. The typical features are that the patient is seen to stare, the eyes may drift upwards and the eyelids flicker. During that time it is apparent that the child is absent (not with you). For a child, recurrent absences of this sort make any form of sustained attention difficult and prevent learning. It is not uncommon for children with absences to visit the doctor with symptoms of inattention and daydreaming, rather than a complaint of seizures themselves.

Complex partial seizures (temporal lobe seizures)

Complex partial seizures arise from the temporal lobe of the brain which is that portion of the brain that lies under the part of the head we call the temple. Occasionally these may arise from the frontal lobe, in the front part of the brain. They may also sometimes be called psychomotor seizures because they may occur together with psychological or psychiatric features. Complex partial seizures represent one of the more difficult types of seizure both to diagnose and to treat. They represent about 40% of all partial seizures and 25% of all seizures.

There are 3 main groups of causes of temporal lobe seizures. The first includes people who have known brain damage from birth, and those who have meningitis, head injuries or other reasons. The second group includes people who have had status epilepticus, possibly associated with febrile convulsions, earlier in their lives. In the third group, no cause can be identified (idiopathic).

The temporal lobe contains an area known as the limbic system in which the heart, blood vessels, respiration and gastrointestinal systems are represented in terms of function. This area also deals with memory and smell. When one considers that all these functions are represented in the temporal lobe, it is hardly surprising that the symptoms of temporal lobe epilepsy can be very varied and difficult to diagnose. Hence the term **complex** partial seizures. Often there are distortions of sensation which may include strange feelings in the stomach, odd smells, hearing voices or music and sometimes there may be visual hallucinations. One of the better known distortions which occurs in temporal lobe seizures is a sensation of familiarity, of having been there before, which is called the deja vu phenomenon. The person will have an abnormal sense of familiarity with a real situation.

There may also be disturbances of speech – not only does the person have difficulty in talking but may make remarks which are quite inappropriate at the time. Certain emotional features such as fear or strangeness may occur, and occasionally giddiness.

Other features may occur if the electrical activity spreads from being a partial seizure and becomes secondarily generalized. The person may then have a tonic–clonic convulsion. A further complicating feature is that unresponsive staring may occur in temporal lobe epilepsy and this may be confused with true absences (petit mal). In complex partial seizures the attacks are more prolonged and may last some minutes; the person may perform familiar actions but in an unusual and repetitive way.

This can sometimes be associated with difficult behaviour or confused speech. These repetitive activities are called 'automatisms'. Such automatisms may also occur in association with absences. Not all complex partial seizures arise from the temporal lobe, although the majority do. Some may arise from the frontal lobes.

Simple partial seizures (focal seizures)

Partial seizures which are focal (involve one part or one side of the body) are quite common in young infants and in adults.

The part of the body affected depends on where the brain abnormality is situated. The areas which seem to be the most sensitive to stimulation are those which represent the index finger, the thumb, the corner of the mouth and the big toe. Thus it is not uncommon for a focal seizure to start in one of these areas. It may then spread around that area and involve that side of the body. Consciousness will be retained unless secondary generalization occurs.

Myoclonic seizures

These are brief, involuntary (carried out subconsciously) contractions of the muscles. Quite often the contractions are symmetrical, most often involving the muscles of the head and upper limbs. The jerks may be rhythmic or sporadic. Sometimes myoclonic seizures may be followed by grand mal seizures.

Other seizure types exist. The main ones have been described above and further information can be obtained from your doctor and/or epilepsy association.

Status epilepticus

This implies a severe continuous seizure or repeated seizures with incomplete recovery of consciousness. The vast majority of fits will stop after a few minutes, but occasionally they will last considerably longer or may occur sufficiently frequently to become a major medical problem. This is status epilepticus.

It is difficult to answer the question so often asked: 'How long can a fit last before it becomes dangerous?' All that one can say is that seizures lasting more than about 30 minutes may be associated with brain damage. Status epilepticus thus represents a medical emergency, so if a seizure lasts more than ten minutes, urgent medical or paramedical assistance should be sought.

What makes a seizure start?

Perhaps surprisingly, this is remarkably difficult to answer. Some people can identify events which precede some, or most, of their seizures. These events include stress, fatigue, alcohol, fever and menstruation (see pages 81–2). However, for most people seizures are quite unpredictable. Indeed this is one of the most irritating things about epilepsy, namely that seizures may occur at any time.

The easiest way to explain the commencement of a seizure is to appreciate that brain cells are normally in a state of balance. Brain cells are subject to positive (excitatory) and negative (inhibitory) influences. Normally these influences are balanced and the brain cells function normally. These influences are mediated by chemicals in the brain. For reasons that we do not fully understand, at various, often unpredictable, times there seem to be chemical changes which alter this finely tuned balance and a seizure may result.

Whilst the brain chemical abnormalities are not yet fully understood, more is known about them now than in the past and it can be hoped that in time it will be possible to devise medications (anticonvulsants) which stop the chemical imbalance from occurring and thus prevent seizures.

Do people have a warning before the start of a fit?

Many people have a warning before the start of a fit. Indeed the warning (aura) may really be considered as part of the fit. An aura is a sensation which precedes loss/alteration of consciousness and is actually the beginning of the seizure. The nature of the aura will depend on the part of the brain in which the seizure begins. For most people the aura is very short indeed and cannot be used to good purpose. For others it may be sufficiently long, for example about a minute, that they can get to a place of safety to have the seizure. For yet other people, there may be sensations or symptoms such as 'being off colour', headache, tummy ache etc. which may last for a day or several days before a seizure. There has been some discussion about the possibility of self hypnosis during an aura to prevent the coming seizure. If this is possible at all, it must (extremely rarely) be a practical proposition.

Can you stop a fit once it has started?

The general answer to this is no. However, having said this there are people with epilepsy who will tell you that they can do just this. Whether the episodes which can be terminated at will are stress related, pseudoseizures or something else is unclear. Observers cannot stop a seizure once it has commenced and should not attempt to restrain someone having a seizure.

If I have a convulsive seizure on my own could I choke?

This is most unlikely. Choking in epilepsy is mistakenly assumed to be due to people swallowing their tongue. This cannot occur; it is a physical impossibility for someone to swallow their tongue. There may be an accumulation of saliva in the mouth, as during a seizure with all the muscular activity going on, it is not always possible to swallow normally. Saliva will spill out of the mouth and may froth leading to the description of 'frothing at the mouth'. The accumulated saliva leads to the choking noises heard during a major seizure. It is for this reason that during a major seizure it is recommended that the person be turned onto their side, allowing the saliva to dribble out of the mouth rather than accumulating in the throat, thus keeping their airway clear.

How long can a febrile convulsion last before doing damage to the brain?

Not surprisingly there is no absolute answer to this question. Most febrile convulsions are brief (a few minutes) and whilst unpleasant and frightening for the parents, are harmless. Occasionally febrile convulsions may be prolonged (more than 30 minutes) and the longer they last, the greater the chance of there being some damage. Having said this, there are people who have had prolonged febrile convulsions lasting several hours who have been quite fine subsequently. On the other hand, there is a known relationship between prolonged febrile convulsions and subsequent temporal lobe epilepsy.

How many febrile convulsions should happen in a day before I call the doctor?

As a general rule it can be said that if more than one febrile convulsion occurs with a single episode of illness this is a matter of some concern and you should contact your doctor at once or go to the closest hospital.

Should I restrain a child who is having a tonic–clonic seizure?

No you should not. Follow the advice on pages 99–100 as to what to do during a major seizure. The person should not be restrained either during or after the seizure. After the seizure some people will be confused and will wander about. Do not restrain them. Simply be with them to ensure that they do not injure themselves. If you attempt to restrain them, in their confused state, they may lash out. This is how the myth of people with epilepsy being aggressive has arisen.

What is photosensitive epilepsy?

This is one of the types of reflex epilepsy; that is, seizures occurring in response to a particular stimulus. There are many different types of reflex epilepsy but photosensitivity is the commonest.

It is usually associated with watching television, more especially getting very close to the set whilst changing channels, computer games (not video display units), flickering lights such as strobe lights or very bright sunlight. It usually commences in late childhood or adolescence and usually stops in the third or fourth decade of life. The seizures are most often tonic–clonic in nature, but there may be myoclonus or atypical absence seizures. In the main, if the provoking factor can be avoided, there is no need for medication. Should medication be required, sodium valproate is the drug of choice.

What is the Lennox–Gastaut syndrome?

The Lennox–Gastaut syndrome is a condition in which there are mixed seizures and for which the outlook, albeit poor, is now reasonably well understood. It is perhaps easiest to understand it as an extension of infantile spasms (West's syndrome) but which occurs in the preschool-aged child. The main features are head nodding, drop attacks and absences.

The condition is frequently associated with mental retardation and brain damage due to a diversity of conditions. The seizures are usually quite difficult to control and the medications of choice are the benzodiazepines (clobazam, clonazepam or nitrazepam) and sodium valproate. There is also a role for steroid medications such as ACTH or prednisone. The outlook both for seizure control and normal intelligence is rather poor.

Because I've damage to the temporal lobe, my neurologist said that I will never gain good seizure control. Is this true?

This is a matter of emphasis. The term 'never' is probably incorrect. In essence, patients with complex partial seizures (temporal lobe epilepsy) exhibit greater difficulty in seizure control than do those persons with the generalized epilepsies (tonic–clonic or absence seizures). Probably only about 50% of those with complex partial seizures will improve significantly with anticonvulsant medication. Remember, however, that 50% *will* improve.

For those patients with intractable complex partial seizures, it is important to look at seizure-provoking factors such as fatigue, stress, alcohol etc., all of which can be modified to some degree. Finally, surgery should be considered (see page 52).

My father has nocturnal epilepsy, but during the day, whilst sleeping, had a seizure. After this he drove his car. Should he have done this?

Firstly, your father has shown that he does not have nocturnal epilepsy as such, but has sleep-associated epilepsy. In other words, he has seizures only when asleep, be this during the day or at night. As to driving his car after a seizure, if he was fully recovered, it should have been quite safe. This, however, is illegal and he should discuss the situation with the Department of Motor Transport (see page 70).

My daughter, aged 8 years, was diagnosed as having absence seizures just before she turned 5 years old. She is not on medication and the only time she has a seizure now is when she is doing her routine piano practice before school. She is a keen student so there is no reluctance on her part to practise and she never appears to have absence seizures at any other time than when she is playing the piano. Is there an explanation for this?

It is difficult to be sure if there is a true explanation. One would need to be certain that she is having true absences and is not simply daydreaming. If these are the real thing, it is just possible that it could be a manifestation of musicogenic epilepsy. This is a rare form of reflex epilepsy, similar to photosensitive epilepsy, but with the stimulus being music as opposed to light.

Whatever the explanation, the episodes seem very minor, are not troublesome and do not warrant medication.

If my seizures have all been at night in bed, will they stay that way?

It is probable that they will, but this cannot be stated with absolute certainty. Why some people with epilepsy have seizures solely at night is unclear. Such people may also have the occasional daytime seizure although this is uncommon.

Most people who have solely night time seizures find them reasonably easy to live with. Indeed some people may be unaware that they have had a seizure, whilst others may notice they are stiff, sore or have bitten their tongue on waking.

My son has temporal lobe epilepsy. He is 7 years old. Lately he is exhibiting overt sexual behaviour, at school and in the neighbourhood. He is running naked outside and has done this at school once. Do you think this behaviour is related to his epilepsy? His seizures are under control at present on Tegretol.

This is a very difficult question to answer. It is possible that this behaviour could be a manifestation of temporal lobe epilepsy. However, as his seizures are well controlled this is unlikely. Pointers suggesting that these could be non-convulsive seizures would be if the episodes begin and end abruptly and if he has no recollection of the episodes. The other possibility is that this is a behavioural trait which he has developed either related to his epilepsy or for some other reason. The only definitive way of determining what these episodes are would be to do an EEG during an episode. This might be difficult, but is not impossible. If during an episode the EEG demonstrates seizure activity, then the episodes are seizures. If not, they are unlikely to be.

Chapter 4
How is Epilepsy Diagnosed and what Tests are Used?

There are numerous tests that can be used to try to diagnose epilepsy. This chapter outlines some of the investigations that your doctor may suggest to you as being worthwhile.

Clinical History

The most important aspect in making a diagnosis of epilepsy is obtaining a good description of the seizures, either from the patient, parent or other people who may have witnessed the fit. Remember that seizures very rarely occur where the doctor can see them, so a good description is all important.

Physical examination

All patients with epilepsy should have a full physical examination the first time they present to their doctor. In primary (idiopathic) epilepsy, physical examination usually reveals no abnormalities. In secondary epilepsy, there may be abnormalities of the nervous system which can be detected.

Laboratory tests

Your doctor may suggest tests which include measuring the blood sugar concentration, blood calcium, magnesium and, rarely, amino acids. It may also, in certain situations, be desirable to look at a child's chromosome pattern. A lumbar puncture, which means obtaining a sample of spinal fluid, is needed in some cases, but is not a routine investigation in epilepsy. It is appropriate if a brain infection (meningitis or encephalitis) is suspected.

Electroencephalography

The electroencephalograph (EEG) measures differences in electrical activity between different parts of the head, arising from the spontaneous activity of the underlying brain cells.

Routine EEG   When your doctor requests an EEG for you, or your child, this entails going to an EEG laboratory where electrodes will be placed on the scalp and connected to an electrical recorder. While the recording takes place, it is important that the subject be relatively still, as any muscular movement may be recorded on the EEG tracing and will make it difficult to interpret. Keeping still can be difficult for children and to get a satisfactory recording from a young child may take well over an hour.

The EEG is regarded by many, parents included, as the mainstay of the diagnosis of epilepsy. While this may be true, it is important to bear in mind that the EEG has very real limitations. These include the fact that from a technical point of view it may be difficult to obtain an adequate recording in a young child. Perhaps more important is the fact that often patterns obtained on an EEG are non-specific. In other words, they suggest that something might be wrong, but do not provide precise information as to what the problem is. Furthermore, it is important to remember that an EEG is recorded over a short period of time, perhaps 20 minutes, so that for the person who has occasional seizures, the brain's electrical activity may be quite normal at the time that the EEG is done. About 40% of patients with epilepsy have a normal EEG and about 15% of non-epileptic persons may have an abnormal EEG. Thus the EEG does not necessarily give the whole answer and indeed sometimes may be quite confusing.

Special EEG studies   Occasionally it may be necessary to do a more sophisticated EEG in patients where there is diagnostic difficulty. Telemetry implies the use of long-term EEG recording techniques, with or without video observation, to allow better definition of complex or ill-explained fits. This is done by obtaining an EEG recording during the actual fit. It is of value in people with complicated epileptic problems.

Computerized tomography (CT scanning)

This is an x-ray procedure in which the patient lies with the head held still in an x-ray machine. A rapid sequence of x-rays of the skull and brain within it are taken and then an injection of dye is given into a vein and the sequences repeated. It is a painless procedure, although young children may be a bit scared by all the machinery. As it is imperative to lie still to get adequate pictures, it may be necessary to give a light general anaesthetic in the very young child.

In primary (idiopathic) epilepsy, the CT scan is often of little help. In less than 10% of persons is any useful information obtained. On the other hand, in secondary epilepsy the CT scan is a lot more useful as the brain damage, or other brain problems, can actually be seen.

PET scanning and MRI

These two techniques, positron emission tomography (PET) and magnetic resonance imaging (MRI), both have the potential to assist in the diagnosis of epilepsy, especially PET scanning. PET scanning is not yet available in Australia. They are very expensive techniques and so are not widely available. This is quite appropriate as these techniques will not be applicable to the majority of people with epilepsy. They will, however, be of use to epileptics with particular problems of diagnosis or if surgery is being contemplated.

What kind of tests are used in the diagnosis of epilepsy?

The most important aspect of making a diagnosis of epilepsy is obtaining a good history and description of the attacks from the patient, relatives or other observers.

The most widely used test is the electroencephalogram (EEG) which records brain waves and is often quite helpful in the diagnosis of epilepsy (see page 23). Occasionally it may be necessary to do more sophisticated EEG studies such as video-telemetry which is a long-term EEG recording whilst observing the patient with a video camera. This allows actual observation of the seizure whilst simultaneously recording the EEG.

It may also be appropriate, under certain circumstances (see page 26), to do computerized tomography (CT scan) of the brain. This may identify a structural abnormality of the brain. Magnetic resonance imaging (MRI scanning) is a newer technique which may be appropriate in certain circumstances, especially if surgical treatment is being considered.

There is in fact a need for but a few tests. Remember that the most important part of making the diagnosis is the information that you give to the doctor in the first place.

If the EEG is normal, is it still possible to have epilepsy?

Yes it is. The EEG is quite a useful test but is not very specific. It only 'makes the diagnosis' in a limited number of types of epilepsy, more especially childhood absence (petit mal), infantile spasms and benign focal epilepsy of childhood. In all other situations it is just part of the jigsaw which goes towards making a diagnosis. About 40% of people with epilepsy have a normal EEG between seizures and about 15% of non-epileptic persons have an abnormal EEG. So you cannot expect the EEG to provide all the answers.

Should you have a CT scan as a routine screen for epilepsy?

This question raises two issues. Firstly, you should not have a routine anything. Tests should only be done if there is a reason and this should be explained by the doctor to the patient prior to doing a test. Secondly, a CT scan does not in itself make a diagnosis of epilepsy; it may provide information as to the cause of epilepsy. The CT scan will identify structural abnormalities of the brain which may, or may not, be the cause of the epilepsy.

CT scanning is not required in all people with epilepsy and is of less value in childhood than in adult life. It is useful when investigating seizures in the first year of life, in older children if they have focal features associated with their seizures and is probably quite generally applicable in adult practice, especially in older patients where brain disease or abnormalities are more likely.

My EEG has been normal so far after four tests. My doctor says the more often I have it done, the more likely it is to come positive. Is this true?

Yes it is true, but only up to a point. As we have discussed already, the routine EEG samples but a short segment of time.

Not surprisingly therefore, between seizures, the EEG is often normal.

The more often one does an EEG, the more samples one is taking so to speak, the greater the chance of finding an abnormality. This has been studied and the results suggests that the yield rises from about 50% to about 85% after three EEGs. How useful this is, is unclear as the diagnosis of epilepsy, while aided by the EEG, is not solely based on EEG findings. The diagnosis is based largely on the clinical history.

A couple of EEGs may therefore be helpful, but more than that, except for a very good reason, is unlikely to be productive.

I had a funny turn about 4 months ago, which on reading around the subject does not sound like a seizure. I subsequently had an EEG which was abnormal, was told that I had epilepsy and was given medication. I have stopped taking the medication as I am uncertain about the diagnosis.

This is a situation which occurs from time to time and exemplifies 3 important points.

Firstly, not all 'turns' or 'episodes' are seizures. Secondly, a single seizure does not make a diagnosis of epilepsy. By definition, epilepsy implies having recurrent seizures. Finally, as we have already discussed in this chapter, simply having an abnormal EEG does not in itself make a diagnosis of epilepsy.

Stopping the medication and not saying, as yet, that you have epilepsy is probably the right way to go. However, medication should always be ceased gradually, preferably with medical advice.

Chapter 5
Drug Treatment of Epilepsy

There are a number of general principles about the management of epilepsy which we will discuss at the beginning of this chapter. These include:

- The fact that about **70% to 75% of people with epilepsy will achieve good seizure control with medical treatment using anticonvulsants**. About 25% of people will not respond very well to anticonvulsants and some may be helped by surgical means. Partial seizures, especially temporal lobe epilepsy, respond less well to medication than do generalized seizures.

- The observation that 60% to 80% of epileptics who can achieve seizure control with anticonvulsant medication (antiepileptic drugs), need only one medication. This is called **monotherapy** (treatment with one medication only).

Naturally there are some epileptics who will need more than one drug, but rarely more than two. As a matter of principle, when someone first starts to take anticonvulsant medication, the dose should be increased relative to the frequency of the fits. **There should be no need for the addition of another medication unless the fits are not controlled (assuming that the patient is really taking the medication) or side effects from the drug arise.** It is really only in these two situations that the addition of another drug is to be recommended. If side effects have occurred, once the second medication has been commenced, the first should be withdrawn.

Medical treatment

The drugs used in the treatment of the various types of epilepsy we have discussed vary according to the seizure type. Some drugs are better for certain seizures than others. It is, however, important to remember that few anticonvulsants are very specific for particular seizures and that **there is a choice of drugs for any**

particular seizure type. The choice may be related to your doctor's experience, the side effects that he or she might anticipate and the way in which you as an individual tolerate a particular medication. The choice of a single drug is therefore not absolute.

Tonic–clonic (Grand mal) seizures Medications used in the treatment of tonic–clonic seizures include carbamazepine, sodium valproate, phenytoin, primidone, phenobarbitone and clonazepam. The order in which the drugs are listed represents some personal bias by the author. Most people would feel that carbamazepine would be effective with the least side effects, but may disagree with the 'preference' listing of the rest of the drugs. It is important for patients to realize that the solution to which drug is best for them may not be a black and white issue. Different doctors may have slightly different approaches to a particular problem.

Absences (petit mal) The drug of choice for this condition is ethosuximide. An excellent alternative is sodium valproate, but its possible liver side effects make it a drug of second choice. In children whose absences are particularly resistant to treatment, clonazepam may be helpful. If tonic–clonic seizures are present as well, sodium valproate is the drug of choice as it covers both seizure types.

Complex partial seizures (temporal lobe epilepsy) Carbamazepine is the drug of choice with phenytoin or sodium valproate being less acceptable alternatives. Clobazam may be a useful adjunct (additional therapy) in some people with temporal lobe seizures.

Simple partial seizures (Focal seizures) Carbamazepine is the drug of choice, followed by phenytoin, sodium valproate or one of the barbiturates.

Reflex epilepsy Drug therapy is not often needed in this condition. Those whose fits are induced by sitting very close to the television should view it from 3 metres away in a well-lit room. In addition, they should not approach the set in order to adjust it or change the channel. An alternative approach is to cover one eye when approaching the television set. If the photosensitivity is induced by sunlight, then polarized sunglasses should be worn. If medication is required, sodium valproate is the drug of choice.

Infantile spasms The treatment of this condition is difficult and the basis of it little understood. The drugs most commonly used are corticosteroid preparations such as corticotrophin (ACTH) and prednisone. An alternative is a group of drugs, the benzodiazepines, of which the most familiar to the general public would be diazepam (Valium). From this particular group of drugs, nitrazepam and clonazepam may be useful in the management of infantile spasms. Sodium valproate may also be used.

Myoclonic and tonic seizures These are perhaps the most difficult forms of seizures to treat. The drugs of choice are probably sodium valproate, nitrazepam, clonazepam, and ACTH. If these have failed in children, the use of a ketogenic diet, which will be discussed later, may be considered.

What is my medication for?

Medications used in the treatment of epilepsy are called anticonvulsants, which mean that they are used 'against seizures'. Anticonvulsants act on the chemicals in the brain and are used to control your seizures, as well as preventing the development of possible further seizures. Anticonvulsants may also prevent the effects of seizures on the brain itself. Anticonvulsant medication thus has several actions of which you need to be aware.

How good is the drug treatment of epilepsy?

Whilst it is not perfect, the answer to this question must be that drug treatment is pretty good and is getting better. It can be anticipated that about 90% of people with epilepsy will derive some benefit from drug treatment. That benefit will vary from person to person.

The drug treatment of epilepsy is a balance between seizure control and drug side effects. Both of these factors vary from individual to individual and thus 'acceptable seizure control' is a very personal matter. Some people would rather have a few more seizures than suffer drug side effects; others may see this quite differently.

Treatment should be started with one drug only (monotherapy) as it is known that 60% to 70% of people with epilepsy will derive significant benefit from such treatment. Should the first drug not be effective, a second drug should be introduced and the first one withdrawn. If the second drug is not effective or fully effective, then it may be necessary for that person to take more than one medication.

What is monotherapy?

Monotherapy means treatment with one drug only. This is an important concept in the management of epilepsy as it has been shown that the advantages of monotherapy are:

1. That it is effective in providing reasonable seizure control in about 60% of people with epilepsy.
2. It avoids any interactions with other drugs.
3. It reduces the side effects so often seen with multiple drug therapy.

Thus monotherapy is often advantageous, but of course cannot be achieved in all patients. There will be some people who have more difficult epilepsy who need to be receiving more than one drug. There are, however, few people who need to take 2 drugs and very few who require 3 or more drugs. Again this is a matter that you should discuss with your doctor.

As a generalization, the more drugs one is taking, the more side effects are likely to be incurred. These are often chronic in nature and are quite frequently not recognized by the patient as being of any great consequence as they have become so used to them over the years. This particularly applies to the areas of mental slowing and dulling, drowsiness and lethargy.

Can anticonvulsants make seizures worse?

Whilst this is unusual, yes they can. Nor do they have to be given in high dosage for this to occur. It has long been known that with excessive phenytoin dosage, seizures may get worse. However it has also become apparent that with other drugs such as diazepam, clobazam, sodium valproate and carbamazepine that occasionally, even in acceptable dosage, seizure control may deteriorate. Why this should occur is unclear.

Another situation where anticonvulsants may make things worse is the person who is taking 3 or 4 medications. The usual setting for this is the person who has difficult epilepsy and who ends up getting one medication after another with little improvement. It has been quite clearly shown that in a good proportion of such people, decreasing the drug load to, shall we say, 2 drugs is often associated with an improvement in seizure control, and very importantly, a general feeling of wellbeing. They feel less dopey and tired, are more alert and show an improvement in memory.

As a generalization, those people with epilepsy who are taking 3 or more anticonvulsants should have the situation reviewed. It may be that they need all those drugs, but it is possible that some of them could manage just as well with at least one drug less and would feel better for it.

If medication is not helping, would it be better to be off it?

This is a difficult question and there is no absolute answer. There are some people with epilepsy who answer this question themselves and simply cease taking their medication **(this should never be done suddenly, but slowly over some months)**. If they do not get any worse, then presumably they are happy with their decision. Should the seizures get worse, they will usually go back onto their medication having satisfied themselves that the medication is in fact of some help. Others do not go the whole hog and stop their medication, but take it sporadically. This really does not answer the question and achieves little. If medication is to be taken, reasonable blood levels must be achieved, which means taking the medication regularly.

Whether to come off medication also depends on the seizure type and thus the risk of what may occur if the seizures get worse. For example for someone with tonic–clonic seizures, the risk of status epilepticus is higher than someone who has partial or complex partial seizures. Occupation also comes into this decision; if having more seizures means a real risk of losing ones job or driving licence, then presumably this would not be a wise thing to do. This is a matter of personal choice.

Whilst there is no absolute answer to this question, it is appreciated that there are some people who feel that their medication is not helping and thus would like to know what they would be like off it. This is a reasonable request which should be discussed in detail with your doctor.

I have tried all the anticonvulsants and there are too many side effects. I am presently taking clobazam but still having seizures. What is the next step?

There are some people who find themselves in this predicament and who ask if they might not be better, or just as badly off, with no medication at all. This is a quite reasonable request and should be considered, if only because some people are so fed up with taking medication with no apparent effect, that they will stop taking it themselves without supervision, which may be dangerous.

There are 3 main reasons why seizures may not come under control. Firstly the person may have particularly resistant epilepsy, secondly they may not take their medication regularly and thus not benefit from treatment and finally the seizures may not be epileptic in nature (pseudoseizures).

For those whose epilepsy is resistant to all medications or in whom side effects are intolerable, the possibility of surgery should be considered, especially for temporal lobe epilepsy (see page 52).

My epilepsy is just 2 blackouts in 18 months. I do not want to take medication and am hoping to become pregnant. Is medication necessary?

This is a difficult question to answer without knowing more about the 'blackouts' and the events surrounding them. It may be that these were not really seizures or that they may have been seizures which were provoked by a trigger factor such as lack of sleep, alcohol etc. (see page 81). In both situations it would be inappropriate to make a diagnosis of epilepsy and medication would be unnecessary. In other words, it is important to be sure that these 2 'blackouts' were in fact epileptic in nature.

Even if they were epileptic in nature, because of the long gap between seizures, some may not feel it warranted to prescribe medication. There is no clear-cut, black and white answer to this sort of problem which really needs to be resolved by common sense discussion between yourself and your doctor.

Should my child continue with anticonvulsants when he is sick and not eating?

The answer to this question is quite definitely **yes**. The reason for being so emphatic is that most childhood illnesses are associated with fever and in turn fever is a provoking factor for seizures. Many parents of children with epilepsy will have noticed that when their child, whose seizures are well controlled, develops an intercurrent illness, often associated with fever, that there is an increase in seizure frequency. This is because fever lowers the seizure threshold and so lets seizures that would otherwise be controlled 'slip through'. In young children, episodes of diarrhoea and vomiting may make the administration of medication difficult. Contact your doctor.

It is therefore particularly important to maintain anticonvulsant treatment during episodes of illness. If the child is unable or unwilling to take the medication and has missed a dose or two, you should contact your doctor at once. It may be necessary for the child to be admitted to hospital for a few days until the illness has subsided.

What if I forget to take my medication?

If you forget to take just one dose once in a while, it probably does not matter. It would be safe to take twice the dose next time to make up for the missed one. This may make you a bit sleepy.

If you are forgetting doses on a regular basis, you need to have a good look at your lifestyle so that you can arrange it better. Most anticonvulsants can be taken twice daily; occasionally it is necessary to take medication 3 times a day. Many people do not like to take medication at work or at school. Thus twice-daily dosage is preferrable. If this is the case, take your medication with breakfast and your evening meal. If you are taking more than one medication it may be helpful to obtain a pill dispenser such as a Dosett which allows you to put your pills out at the start of the week. Using this system, if the pills are still in the container, then you have not taken them. This acts as a reminder to take your pills and it also answers the common question 'Did I take my medication this morning?' If it is not in the dispenser, you did; if it is still in the dispenser, you did not.

How can I tell if my child is under or over medicated?

If your child is under medicated, he or she will continue to have seizures. In other words, they are not taking sufficient medication to control the seizures. This comment is valid irrespective of the amount of medication that a person is taking. Some people will have mild epilepsy and need little medication, whilst others will have more severe epilepsy and need more medication. People vary in the rate at which they metabolize (break down) anticonvulsants in their body and this also affects their dosage requirements.

In the main, when over-medicated with anticonvulsants, there will be drowsiness, lethargy and often a general slowing down. Sometimes in children, there may be an increase in activity, perhaps even hyperactivity associated with over-medication and there may be an increase in seizure frequency.

You need to be aware of the side effects of the medication(s) that you or your child are taking. By knowing this, you will be aware when over-medication occurs. (See Chapter 19).

What will happen if I forget my tablets and I am staying away from home?

Ideally, this should not happen! However if it does, from a practical point of view, it depends on how long you will be away. If it is just an overnight stay and you miss one or two doses, you may well get away with it. If it is a weekend or longer, go to a hospital, doctor or chemist. Tell them 'I have epilepsy and take medication X which I left at home. May I have enough tablets to tide me over the next few days?'

Are anticonvulsants addictive?

The answer to this is yes and no depending upon how you define addiction and which anticonvulsant you are taking. It is well known that people with epilepsy who have been on medication for some time, may have withdrawal seizures if they come off the medication suddenly or rapidly. This probably does not represent addiction as such, but may be verging on it.

On the other hand, some people who have come off the barbiturates and some of the benzodiazepines (particularly clonazepam), especially if they have done so rapidly, will have suffered a withdrawal reaction. This reaction is identical to that seen when coming off recognized addictive drugs with anxiety, agitation, fear, palpitations, perspiration, etc. This form of reaction can be minimized, or avoided, by coming off a particular medication slowly over 3 to 9 months.

These comments imply that there is an addictive component potentially associated with long-term barbiturate or benzodiazepine usage, but not with the other anticonvulsants.

I'm really scared of having a seizure. Can I increase my medication to avoid this?

Seizure control is a balance between the number of seizures and drug side effects. All anticonvulsant medications have side effects to a greater or lesser extent. Certainly you can increase your medication, but if you are drowsy and wobbly on your feet, you may be worse off than having the occasional seizure.

This balance is a very individual one which you, the person with epilepsy, must decide upon. It is often achieved by trial and error. Discuss it with your doctor and if necessary, ask to be referred to a specialist in epilepsy. What may be suitable for you in the way of medication may well not be ideal for someone else. You need to be treated as an individual and this may necessitate some experimentation with medications and dosages. You also need to contact your epilepsy association to have a good chat about your epilepsy, accepting it and coming to grips with it.

Should I expect any withdrawal symptoms when coming off my anticonvulsants?

When coming off the barbiturates, clonazepam, diazepam and to a lesser extent phenytoin, withdrawal symptoms can certainly occur. This is not the case with carbamazepine and sodium valproate.

Withdrawal symptoms can be minimized by coming off the drug slowly over 3 to 9 months. Despite this some people will still have withdrawal symptoms. If anticonvulsants have to be withdrawn rapidly, this should be done in hospital to deal with the withdrawal reaction and the possibility of rebound seizures.

Withdrawal symptoms should not be confused with the considerable anxiety which some people suffer at the thought of coming off medication and losing their 'security blanket'. The fear of having another seizure, especially after having been seizure free for some years, is very real for many people coming off medication. This is something they need to discuss with their local epilepsy association and/or their doctor.

Chapter 6
Drug Interactions and Side Effects

The medications used in the treatment of epilepsy (anticonvulsants) are all quite potent medications which act on the brain to prevent seizures. Not surprisingly with such medications there may be some unwanted side effects. It is important that you be aware of the possible side effects of any medication that you are taking so that you can report it to your doctor (see Chapter 19). In addition, if you are taking more than one medication, the medications may interact in your body to produce side effects or one medication may affect the way in which another medications works. There are not many important interactions which relate to anticonvulsants, but you should know about those which affect your medication(s); refer to Table 2 and ask your doctor.

Do all anticonvulsant drugs have side effects?

The answer is yes. This of course applies not only to anticonvulsants but to all drugs. All drugs have the potential to produce side effects; some more frequently than others and in addition some people are more susceptible to side effects than others. That is why not everyone taking a particular drug develops side effects.

With respect to anticonvulsants, each drug has a number of side effects, some more striking than others (see Chapter 19). It is important that you be aware of the side effects of the medication(s) that you are taking. It is up to your doctor to discuss these with you and it is up to you to ask about them. Many people do not have any side effects, but for those who do, it is important that they discuss these with their doctor.

Does medication affect my memory?

Yes it may. For most people with epilepsy this does not appear to be a major problem, but for some it is a very irritating part of

Anticonvulsants	Drugs to Avoid	Explanation
Carbamazepine	Erythromycin (antibiotic) Chloramphenicol (antibiotic) Cimetidine (anti-ulcer agent)	These drugs slow the breakdown of carbamazepine in the body and lead to its accumulation and toxicity.
Clobazam	None recorded	
Clonazepam	None recorded	
Ethosuximide	None of note	
Nitrazepam	None recorded	
Phenytoin	Chloramphenicol (antibiotic) Cimetidine (anti-ulcer agent) Isoniazid (anti-TB drug)	These drugs slow the breakdown of phenytoin in the body and lead to it's accumulation and toxicity.
	Aspirin	Aspirin can displace phenytoin from plasma proteins and lead to toxicity.
Phenobarbitone Primidone	None of note	Phenobarbitone and primidone may lower the blood levels of other anticonvulsants and render them less effective.
Sodium Valproate	None of note	Sodium valproate can displace phenytoin from plasma proteins and lead to toxicity.

Table 2. *Common drug interactions with anticonvulsants. First look at the left hand column (the anticonvulsants which you may be taking) and then the next column, which are the drugs to avoid. Trade names of the drugs are given in Appendix 2.*

their epilepsy. It is not uncommon for people with epilepsy to complain of a poor or deteriorating memory. There are a number of factors which are involved in this which include the person's basic memory capabilities, brain disease, attention difficulties, seizure frequency and drug therapy. Memory is worse with early seizure onset, the greater the frequency of fits, the longer the duration of uncontrolled epilepsy and the greater the total number of lifetime fits.

With respect to the effects of medication, it would appear that memory is more affected in persons taking the 'older generation' of anticonvulsants (phenytoin, the barbiturates and clonazepam) than those taking other anticonvulsants. A change in anticonvulsants, if possible, may be worthy of consideration.

Do anticonvulsants change personality or does epilepsy do this?

It used to be said that there was such a thing as an 'epileptic personality'. This is no longer accepted. Certainly people with epilepsy have varied personalities as do others in society, but there is no clear-cut, identifiable 'epileptic personality'. The issue is sometimes slightly confused, as a proportion of those with epilepsy are brain damaged and for that reason may have unusual personalities. It is probable that frequent seizures over prolonged periods may alter intellectual functioning and could also modify personality. In a study conducted in 1984 it has been shown that adults with epilepsy quite commonly have psychosocial problems which are emotional, interpersonal, vocational and financial in nature. These issues need to be considered in the management of the 'whole person' with epilepsy.

Of some importance are the effects that anticonvulsants can have on what is called 'higher cerebral function' which includes memory, learning, behaviour and so on. **It is now generally accepted that the older generation of anticonvulsants including phenytoin and the barbiturates, as well as clonazepam, have a greater effect on learning and memory than do the newer drugs (carbamazepine, sodium valproate and clobazam).** With all the anticonvulsants it is possible that a proportion of children will become overactive and behaviourally difficult, especially with phenobarbitone and clonazepam.

My son has epilepsy and takes sodium valproate. He has bad temper tantrums. Are these related to the epilepsy or the drug?

When thinking about this sort of problem it is important to bear in mind that many children have temper tantrums. Indeed they are commoner than is epilepsy. In other words your child may well have had temper tantrums if he did not have epilepsy. In fact this is the likeliest possibility. A further factor to be taken into account is that epileptic children are known to have more behavioural problems than children without epilepsy and also are more overprotected by their parents. This may also account for the temper tantrums.

It is most unlikely that the temper tantrums relate to the epilepsy as such. Whilst it is possible for people with complex partial seizures (temporal lobe epilepsy) to have outbursts of rage, this is uncommon, especially in childhood. Sodium valproate, like many of the anticonvulsants, can sometimes make children irritable and overactive, but would very rarely cause the sort of outbursts described here.

Do I have to put up with this double vision?

The answer to this is quite obviously no. Double vision is usually related to excessive drug dosage, especially with carbamazepine or phenytoin. In this situation it would be appropriate to check the blood levels of the medication and if they are unusually high, to reduce the dosage. In some people, the blood levels may be within the so-called therapeutic range, but they still have double vision. This is probably because they are unusually sensitive to the drug and again the dosage should be reduced.

Occasionally the double vision may relate to the underlying problem such as a head injury or may occur after brain surgery in which case little can be done about it. However drug-induced causes should always be sought as these are correctable.

Can sodium valproate cause obesity?

Yes it can, but so can most of the other anticonvulsants. Why this occurs is unclear although it is probably related, to some degree, to brain stimulation of appetite as most people who put on weight state that they are eating more. Such weight gain is seen especially with sodium valproate, clobazam and to a lesser extent carbamazepine. It can however occur with any of the other anticonvulsants.

The frequency of this side effect is uncertain but with sodium valproate is reported as occurring in 1% to 5% of persons, especially if they are taking sodium valproate with another anticonvulsant. The weight gain can sometimes be quite dramatic with an increase of up to 20% of the previous body weight. The reported incidence with clobazam varies from about 1% to 10%. This drug-induced weight gain is often quite difficult to manage, but requires food restriction and increased exercise. It usually recedes on coming off the drug, but this may take some long time.

My son has infantile spasms and is taking clonazepam. He drools a lot. What does this mean?

Clonazepam is one of the benzodiazepine group of drugs which includes other agents such as clobazam, nitrazepam and diazepam. It is a property of this group of drugs to increase some secretions. This is especially the case with clonazepam which quite frequently leads to increased salivation and drooling. It may also increase secretion in the lungs which can be a problem in handicapped children who are immobile as this can lead to mucus plugging and subsequent chest infection.

If I am sick, can I take painkillers?

When taking any medications, it is important to be aware of any interactions that may occur with other medications. This applies as much to people with epilepsy as to those with any other chronic condition requiring medical treatment. There are many interactions between drugs, but most are very uncommon indeed. The common ones that affect anticonvulsants are shown in Table 2.

It is quite safe to take painkillers with anticonvulsant medications with paracetamol perhaps being preferred to aspirin.

My child is aggressive and hyperactive. How much of this is due to his condition or his medication?

This is a common question which is often difficult to answer. Probably the most important aspect is comparing the child's behaviour before treatment to that since receiving treatment. If the behaviour is worse, why?

There may be several reasons for this. The child's own personality may contribute to the behaviour, it may be exacerbated by the medications and occasionally it may be related to the epilepsy itself. The latter is actually quite uncommon. Occasionally, the patient with temporal lobe epilepsy may exhibit aggression and have bursts of overactivity. Some medications, especially barbiturates, clonazepam and phenytoin, are liable to cause overactivity. The other anticonvulsants, carbamazepine, sodium valproate and clobazam may also have this effect, but usually to a lesser extent.

I have become really moody and depressed. Is that the medication?

Assuming that these symptoms have occurred since going onto the medication, then it is possible that they may be related to the medication. The 'older generation' of anticonvulsants (phenytoin, barbiturates and clonazepam) are more likely to produce effects on mood, attention, memory and learning than the 'newer' agents (carbamazepines, sodium valproate, clobazam). These effects may be related simply to taking the medication, whilst in other persons the effects may be a manifestation of over-medication. It may be appropriate to check the anticonvulsant blood level and/or consider changing to another anticonvulsant.

Some people may become moody, anxious or depressed as a reaction to their epilepsy. This is not uncommon and needs to be recognized and dealt with.

Should being on carbamazepine cause me to have period pains?

The answer to this question is probably no. However, it does allow brief discussion of the effect of anticonvulsants on oral contraception. Most of the regular anticonvulsants (carbamazepine, phenytoin and the barbiturates) speed up the way in which the liver breaks down drugs and other compounds in the body. **This means that the oral contraceptive is broken down more rapidly in the body and is thus less effective. The risk of 'pill failure' is not inconsiderable.**

It is common practice these days to prescribe low-dose oral contraceptives. With the abovementioned anticonvulsants because of their effect on the liver, a low-dose pill is likely to be ineffectual. A high-dose oral contraceptive or another form of contraception should be used.

My baby seems to be having more seizures since she went onto medication. Could the medication be causing the seizures? What should I do about it?

The medication is not causing the seizures, but it may be making them worse. It is not often appreciated that in some people, fortunately very few, all the anticonvulsants may make seizures worse.

This can occur in two settings. Firstly with phenytoin and carbamazepine, excessive dosage leading to drug intoxication may be associated with an increase in seizure frequency. The second situation is an unpredictable response in which, with normal dosage, there may be a deterioration in seizure control. This latter response is usually seen with sodium valproate and the benzodiazepines (diazepam, nitrazepam, clonazepam and clobazam). When deterioration in seizure control occurs it usually does so quite soon (days or weeks) after the drug has been introduced.

If this does occur, consult your doctor at once to discuss this situation. It may be necessary either to check the drug blood levels or withdraw the recently introduced medication.

My son's liver function is down according to latest tests. The paediatrician says it is down more than last time, but not to worry. He is on sodium valproate and carbamazepine. Should he come off sodium valproate? What are the signs to look for, in case there is any problem with the liver?

Many drugs, and most anticonvulsants, alter liver function as measured in the blood. The test looks at what are called liver enzymes which are often elevated as a result of an effect of the drug on the liver tissue. With anticonvulsants, a mild elevation of liver enzymes is so very common as to be essentially normal. Indeed it may be regarded as part and parcel of taking an anticonvulsant.

On the other hand, most of the anticonvulsants can very occasionally be associated with liver damage. The drug of greatest concern is sodium valproate, although serious liver toxicity is excessively rare. Rather than performing liver function tests regularly, as they are not very helpful, it is better for people to be aware of the symptoms of liver damage. These include a flu-like feeling, tenderness in the liver area, often an increase in seizures and finally jaundice (yellowness of the whites of the eyes). If these occur, contact your doctor immediately.

Chapter 7
Blood Level Measurements

Patients with epilepsy will be familiar with the practice of having blood samples taken from time to time to measure the blood levels of their anticonvulsant drugs. When a drug is administered to a person, it accumulates in the body over a few days and eventually reaches a certain level in the bloodstream. As far as anticonvulsants are concerned, after taking medication regularly for about a week, the blood concentration will be at what is called 'steady state'. If the patient continues to take the medication regularly thereafter, while there may be slight ups and downs in the concentration (level) over a 24-hour period, it will eventually remain stable (at a steady state).

Therapeutic drug monitoring determines whether the patient's blood level is within what is called the 'therapeutic range' (see Fig. 2). This is the range of blood concentrations within which the majority of people with epilepsy will have good seizure control with minimal drug side effects. This does not mean that every patient **has** to be within the therapeutic range. Some patients may have their symptoms controlled very well with their blood levels below the therapeutic range, while others, if they do not have side effects may need to be above the therapeutic range. The therapeutic range is just an average level. However, the therapeutic range and blood level monitoring are very useful for the doctor for some anticonvulsants, especially phenytoin. Blood level measurements may sometimes be useful for carbamazepine, phenobarbitone, primidone and perhaps ethosuximide. **They are of little, if any, value for sodium valproate, nitrazepam, clonazepam or clobazam.**

When should blood levels be measured?

Unfortunately, it has become almost routine to measure the blood levels of anticonvulsants in all epileptic patients, every

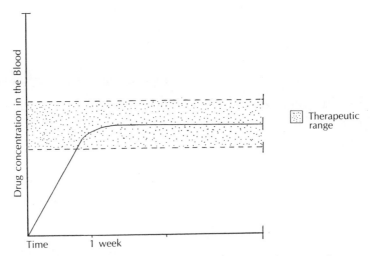

Figure 2.   *After about a week of taking medication regularly, a steady state is reached. If the medication is taken regularly thereafter, the blood concentration remains fairly constant. The therapeutic range is the range of blood concentrations of anticonvulsant drugs within which most patients have good seizure control.*

time they visit their doctor. **This is quite unnecessary and has almost replaced conversation with the doctor which is so essential to those who have epilepsy.** Obviously, if a patient has good seizure control and no side effects, there is little need to measure any blood levels. **The indications for blood level monitoring include:**

Poor seizure control   This may be because the person is not taking his or her medication (non-compliance), is not receiving a sufficient amount of an appropriate medication or is receiving an inappropriate medication. It may also be because the fits are uncontrollable, that the diagnosis of epilepsy is in fact wrong or that there has been a sudden increase in seizures.

Polytherapy   This describes patients who are receiving more than one drug, usually because their seizures are difficult to control. There may be interactions between the drugs and in that case measuring the blood levels may be of value.

Side effects   If a patient is taking only one drug (monotherapy) and has side effects, there may be no need to measure the blood level as it will be obvious what the cause is. It may be sufficient to stop the drug for a day or two to let the blood level decline. On the other hand if a patient is receiving several drugs (polytherapy), it may not be possible to know which drug is causing the problem without measuring the blood levels.

In the very young, the elderly or the handicapped   These groups may handle anticonvulsants differently in the body and may not be able to describe side effects which they are experiencing.

Phenytoin   Phenytoin is broken down in the body by the liver in a rather complicated way which is different to other anticonvulsants. The difficulty with phenytoin is that, contrary to expectation, as the dosage is increased the concentration in the blood stream does not increase proportionally (see Fig. 3). This means that as the dosage is increased, the blood concentration may suddenly rise quite rapidly and the patient may become intoxicated. For this reason, patients who are receiving phenytoin should have regular blood tests, at least when they are being started on treatment, until they are stabilized on the medication.

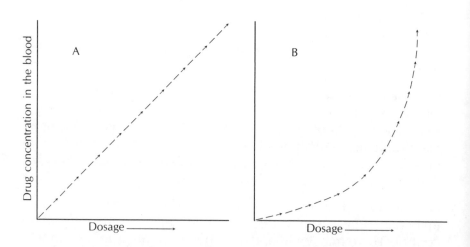

Figure 3.   *For most anticonvulsants, as the dose is increased, the blood concentration rises proportionally (A). However, this is not the case for phenytoin. Sketch B shows the rapid rise in the blood concentration for a very small increase in dosage of phenytoin.*

What does blood level monitoring do?

Blood level monitoring of anticonvulsants has become very common practice. Indeed it is probably overdone and has almost become a substitute for conversation with the patient. Its purpose is to make changes in drug dosage that will allow an improvement of seizure control and/or the avoidance of side effects. **By definition therefore, if seizures are well controlled and there are no side effects of note, there is no great purpose in measuring the blood level.** There should be no such concept as 'routine' blood level monitoring. Tests should only be done when there is a good reason for doing them, not just because you happen to call in to see your doctor for a chat or to collect a prescription.

Blood level monitoring is especially useful in people taking phenytoin because of the way in which that drug is handled in the body. This unusual way in which the drug is handled makes finding the correct dose for an individual more difficult than with other anticonvulsants. Thus it is useful to monitor the blood levels whilst the person is being stabilized on the drug. This is not as necessary with the other anticonvulsants but may sometimes be of use for the barbiturates and carbamazepine. Blood level monitoring is of almost no value in people taking sodium valproate, clobazam or clonazepam as there is no good relationship between the blood level and the degree of seizure control.

Other reasons for measuring blood levels of anticonvulsants include: poor seizure control, especially if the person is taking more than one drug, unexplained side effects, during pregnancy and sometimes in children as they are growing and may need dosage changes.

If your doctor measures your blood level every time you go to see him/her, you might care to ask why? Unless it is being done for a definable reason, it is not likely to be serving any great purpose. **Ask questions, don't be subjected to unnecessary tests.**

My son aged 10 takes carbamazepine. His fits are well controlled. He has blood level tests every 3 months. Is this necessary?

Probably not. As discussed at the beginning of this chapter, there must be a reason for doing a blood level test. One could perhaps accept an annual test in a growing child whose seizures are well controlled. You might ask your doctor why the tests are being done.

Different doctors have given me different opinions as to the value of measuring sodium valproate blood levels. What is the position?

Whilst opinions do differ, most people would feel that measuring blood levels of sodium valproate is of little value as there is not a good relationship between the blood level and the degree of seizure control. The reasons for this are complex, but well documented.

As a generalization, it is of little value to measure sodium valproate blood levels unless one suspects that the patient is not taking their medication in which case a very low blood level would be found. In addition, in patients taking high-dose sodium valproate, drowsiness and confusion may occur. If the blood level is very high, the dose should be reduced.

Others would argue that it is worth checking what the level is, to see whether the dose needs to be increased to achieve seizure control. It has been proposed that if the level is above 700μmol/L that a further dose increase will be of no benefit and another anticonvulsant should be tried.

My doctor sent me for a 'free' drug level recently. What does this mean?

All drugs are bound in the blood to proteins. The degree of binding varies from drug to drug. That which is bound to protein is called the 'bound fraction' and that which is not bound is the 'free fraction'. The free fraction is the active component of the drug.

When measuring blood levels, both the bound and free fractions are measured, giving a 'total' drug level. This is what is measured when you have a blood level done.

In some drugs which are highly bound (90%), other drugs and intercurrent illnesses may alter the binding so that it falls. This means that there is more free drug available, and as this is the active part of the drug, drug toxicity may occur. In this setting, if 'total' drug is measured, the increased free component will not be detected.

The only anticonvulsant for which 'free' drug monitoring is applicable is phenytoin. Even then it is very rarely required. It may be appropriate in those who are malnourished, have liver or kidney disease or are taking drugs such as aspirin or Valium.

Chapter 8
Surgical Treatment of Epilepsy

Surgery is useful for a small proportion of people with epilepsy, mainly those with temporal lobe epilepsy. Even in this group of patients, surgery should only be considered if the seizures cannot be controlled by medication and if the seizures arise from one side of the brain.

Can epilepsy be treated by surgery?

The surgical treatment of epilepsy has been around for some decades and is currently being used more often than in the past. There are 2 main surgical approaches.

1. Procedures in people with intractable, major seizures where surgery is used to either remove an area of brain tissue or cut brain pathways (corpus callosectomy) to stop the seizures spreading within the brain. These approaches are used to improve the quality of life of the person with intractable seizures, rather than to 'cure' the epilepsy.

2. Procedures such as temporal lobectomy (removing a part of the temporal lobe) in persons with temporal lobe epilepsy who have not responded to anticonvulsant treatment. Careful and quite prolonged preoperative assessment is required which will allow exact definition of that area of the temporal lobe from which the seizures arise. For a number of reasons, some people will be found not to be suitable for surgery. Of those who undergo temporal lobectomy, it can be anticipated that about 60% will be seizure free subsequently although most will need to continue taking an anticonvulsant, often in a smaller dose than before.

Surgery certainly does have a role in the management of epilepsy, albeit a limited one.

I am 24 years old and have had temporal lobe epilepsy for 6 years. I have daily seizures despite medication. Should I consider surgery?

Yes you should **consider** it. Before going any further your specialist would want to make sure that you have had a fair trial of all the appropriate anticonvulsants. If so, then you may wish to proceed to being tested for surgery.

This means trying to find out:

● Where your epilepsy is coming from? In other words, where is the epileptic focus within the brain.
● Whether you have a single focus or more than one.
● What your psyche and memory would be like if the affected part of your brain were removed.

To achieve this you would need to be in hospital to have very detailed tests over a 3-week to 3-month period. The tests include detailed EEG studies, CT and MRI scans and detailed psychological testing.

As a broad generalization, if the test showed a single focus in a part of the temporal lobe which could be removed without causing damage, then you would be a surgical candidate. If, on the other hand, you had a focus on both sides of the brain, removing one would probably not help.

My son is 15 years old. He is handicapped and has severe, frequent drop attacks. Despite wearing a helmet he has injured his face and teeth many times. I saw on television about an operation that might help him. What is it?

The operation is called a 'corpus callosectomy' which means dividing about one half of the corpus callosum.

The corpus callosum is a bundle of fibres which connects the two halves of the brain. When this is divided, the seizures do not spread from one side of the brain to the other. The operation may reduce the number of seizures and/or make them milder.

It is not an operation that would ever be considered lightly, but may improve the quality of life of those with incapacitating seizures, especially drop attacks.

Chapter 9
Alternative Medicine and Epilepsy

Many people with epilepsy will from time to time feel fed up and irritated with their epilepsy and/or their medication. At such times they may look at alternative approaches including:

Hypnosis

There is little place for hypnosis in the management of epilepsy. The only exception is the patient who has a long warning (aura) prior to the seizure. If the aura lasts long enough, it is possible to teach the patient self-hypnosis and it is conceivable that the patient may be able to prevent the seizure. This is hardly ever the case, however. The role of hypnosis in reducing stress and thus seizure frequency has not been formally studied.

Naturopathy

Naturopaths feel that epilepsy is due to a deficiency of the B group of vitamins and possibly zinc. Some success is reported in absences (petit mal) but less so in other forms of epilepsy.

Acupuncture

The role of acupuncture in the management of epilepsy is controversial. Acupuncturists see epilepsy as a liver problem because they feel the liver controls muscular rigidity. There is no good evidence that acupuncture helps people with epilepsy.

Dietary treatment

For patients with myoclonic epilepsy or infantile spasms who have failed to respond to respond to medication, the use of a ketogenic diet may be of value. This diet, which is not very palatable, acts by increasing the blood concentration of a variety of acids in the body which, it is suggested, results in some chemical changes in the brain. This may reduce the tendency for brain cells to discharge and also prevent the spread of discharges within the brain. Most people who have been heavily involved in treating children with epilepsy will have had occasional success with this form of treatment. However, taking into account all patients who have been treated with a ketogenic diet, the results have been disappointing.

Are there alternatives to drug therapy?

Certain people, especially those with temporal lobe epilepsy, may be suitable for surgical treatment of their epilepsy. This is called a temporal lobectomy. There are a number of other surgical procedures which may be considered for people with intractable seizures (see page 52).

There does not appear to be any role for so-called 'alternative' therapies. This is not said in a sour grapes fashion, but because there is no proof that any of these therapies are effective. This applies to acupuncture, naturopathy, homeopathy and chiropractic, but not to the ketogenic diet.

Despite this advice, people will still try 'alternative' therapies. That's fine provided that you can be sure that the therapy will not do any harm and also that **you continue your medication** whilst you are trying the new treatment. For some people, it may work for reasons that we do not understand.

Do acupuncture or naturopathy help with seizure control?

The role of acupuncture in the management of epilepsy is controversial. Acupuncturists see epilepsy as being a liver problem because they feel that the liver controls muscular rigidity. There is no good evidence that acupuncture helps people with epilepsy.

Naturopaths believe that epilepsy is due to deficiency of the B group of vitamins and possibly zinc. Some success is reported in absences (petit mal) but less so in other forms of epilepsy.

The reality of the situation is that many people with a chronic problem, be it epilepsy, asthma, backache or headaches, will get fed up with their present treatment and want to try something else. This is quite understandable. With epilepsy, there is no harm in trying these remedies, provided that you do not stop taking your regular medication. Doing so may be dangerous.

Does biofeedback help in epilepsy?

Because of the sudden onset of most seizures, techniques such as biofeedback cannot be effectively employed. It may however be useful in those few people who have an aura of reasonable duration, such as 15 to 30 minutes.

Perhaps more importantly this question raises the issue of the relationship between stress and seizures. It is unlikely that stress as such actually starts epilepsy. However, there is no doubt that stress makes seizures worse at least for some people. This is a very difficult area to study as stress varies so much from person to person. What is stressful for one person may not be for another. However there is growing evidence that paying attention to commonsense lifestyle issues, stress avoidance (as best possible) and an understanding of relaxation may be very useful indeed in reducing seizure frequency. This is an aspect of epilepsy management which does not receive the recognition which it deserves.

Will vitamins help in epilepsy?

At the time of writing, the answer is no. Some patients who have been taking phenytoin and/or barbiturates for many years may become deficient in folic acid and can develop an anaemia. This may need to be treated with folic acid which usually has no effect on seizure control but may very occasionally make seizures worse.

There have been some preliminary studies suggesting that vitamin E may be of some value in people with difficult epilepsy and very frequent seizures. It should be stressed that these studies are preliminary and the effect of vitamin E remains unproven. Pyridoxine and Biotin may have a role to play in some rare seizure disorders of infancy, but are of no value in older children or adults.

What is the relationship between zinc and seizures?

Probably nothing. The only good evidence of any relationship is that a few patients taking sodium valproate developed a skin rash associated with zinc deficiency. The rash responded to zinc supplementation. This has been seen in but a handful of people taking sodium valproate.

Chapter 10
Epilepsy and Children

Epilepsy is very much a childhood disorder with 60% to 70% of epilepsy beginning in childhood. It is especially important that epilepsy in a developing child be well managed so as to avoid possible social, psychological and educational problems. If these issues are not well managed from the outset, they may end up being more troublesome than the actual seizures.

Children should be encouraged to lead full, normal lives (see Chapter 13). Parents and teachers need to be well informed about epilepsy so that they can give the child the best chances possible. Drug doses need to be kept as low as possible whilst still achieving optimal seizure control.

The child needs, with the passage of time, to understand about his/her epilepsy and medications so that they take responsibility for their own condition as they move into the turbulent time of adolescence.

Is sleepwalking associated with epilepsy?

No it is not. Some people with complex partial seizures (temporal lobe epilepsy) may wander around in a confused state, but this is unlikely to be mistaken for sleepwalking.

How can I tell if my child is throwing a temper tantrum or having a seizure because he does both?

As a general rule, temper tantrums occur in response to something which provokes this response. Usually, the child has been chastised or has been forbidden to do something. In other words, there is usually an identifiable provoking factor for temper tantrums. Moreover, they can usually be seen to be 'building up or coming on' and once the episode is over, cease gradually.

58

This is in distinction to episodes of temper associated with epilepsy. This may occur, though uncommonly, in temporal lobe epilepsy. These episodes, like all seizures, begin and end abruptly.

There may be some difficulty in differentiating the seizures from temper tantrums, but with a good history, sometimes aided by EEG studies, it should not be too hard to do.

My 4-year-old daughter has been taking phenobarbitone for 3 months. She has become aggressive and beastly. What can I do?

All the anticonvulsants can have this effect, some more so than others. The worst offender is phenobarbitone which may have this effect in up to 40% of children. The solution is to change to carbamazepine or sodium valproate. The same might occur with these drugs, but the chances are very much less than with phenobarbitone.

My 3-year-old son has been diagnosed as having the Lennox-Gastaut syndrome. He has lots of fits and seems retarded. I am devastated, 6 months ago he was a normal child.

The features of the Lennox-Gastaut Syndrome have been mentioned on page 20. It is a form of myoclonic epilepsy, the cause of which is unknown.

It is an especially distressing condition for parents as they see a normal child develop difficult to control seizures and go backwards intellectually. The distress is made worse by the lack of information about this condition, the difficulty in obtaining seizure control and its poor outlook.

There are a number of treatment options including sodium valproate, steroids (ACTH or prednisone) and benzodiazepines (clobazam, clonazepam, nitrazepam). In many children, the myoclonus improves but may well be replaced by other seizure types (generalized seizures). Some degree of intellectual retardation is almost invariable.

Chapter 11
Epilepsy and Women

Women with epilepsy are quite often concerned about getting pregnant. There appear to be five reasons for this concern. They wish to know:

- if they are likely to hand their epilepsy onto their children;
- whether their seizures will get worse during pregnancy;
- whether it is safe for the baby that the mother should take anticonvulsants drugs during pregnancy;
- if there will be any problems in the newborn baby from these drugs;
- if they can safely breast feed the baby.

With regard to handing on epilepsy to one's children – as mentioned earlier, if one parent has epilepsy, the chances of one of the children having epilepsy are no greater than in the population at large. If both parents have generalized epilepsy, it would appear that the risk of a child having epilepsy is about 10 per cent. So in fact the chance of a child inheriting epilepsy is negligible.

As far as seizures during pregnancy are concerned, the situation is not as clear as it might be. There is evidence that for some women, seizure control may deteriorate, while for others there may in fact be no change or even an improvement.

As a general working rule, it is suggested that people who have more than one tonic–clonic seizure a month are those who are most likely to have a deterioration in seizure control during pregnancy. The deterioration, if it occurs, is most likely during the first three months of pregnancy. There are a number of theories why this may happen, but none have been proved. It may be of value to check the blood anticonvulsant levels during pregnancy, especially if there is a deterioration in seizure control. The blood levels may fall, necessitating an increase in dosage during the pregnancy.

The main concern for parents is whether the anticonvulsants can harm the unborn baby (fetus). It is known by most people with epilepsy that this is a potential hazard. The effects include physical abnormalities in the baby, a process known as **teratogenesis**. Abnormalities have been reported in the offspring of mothers on all the commonly used anticonvulsants with the exception of carbamazepine. This is particularly applicable to phenytoin, barbiturates and sodium valproate. Babies born to mothers who have been on carbamazepine have not been shown to have any physical abnormalities, but may have a smaller head size than other babies. This has not been shown to be any handicap to the babies who have been followed up for 5 years.

The risk of abnormalities in the baby is difficult to assess, but it seems to be most common in mothers on polytherapy (receiving numerous drugs), especially if they are taking 3 or more anticonvulsants. The risk in mothers on phenytoin, with or without other medications, appears to be about a 4% chance of the baby showing features of the 'fetal hydantoin' syndrome. This syndrome consists of cleft palate, abnormalities of the fingers, possible heart abnormalities and mild mental retardation. Thus, at present, it would seem wise to try to change patients over to carbamazepine before conception. This may not be possible in all patients and, of course, many women will first visit their doctor when already pregnant, at which time there is no purpose in making the change.

Anticonvulsants taken by the mother during pregnancy may have some effects on the baby immediately after birth, as they are transmitted to the baby across the placenta. These include the possibility of a mild bleeding tendency and some drowsiness. In mothers who have been taking barbiturates, the infant may occasionally show features of a withdrawal reaction with irritability, jitteriness and poor sucking. None of these features is either common or serious.

As far as breast feeding is concerned, all the anticonvulsant drugs appear in breast milk to some extent. At worst they may produce some mild drowsiness in the baby. There is no reason for mothers with epilepsy not to breast feed if they wish to do so. If the mother is concerned that she might have a fit and drop the baby, she should breast feed sitting on the floor.

Anticonvulsants and the contraceptive pill?

This is an important question for women with epilepsy. Most of the anticonvulsant drugs, with the probable exception of clobazam and sodium valproate, increase the rate at which the liver turns over other drugs which it metabolizes (inactivates). As the oral contraceptive pill is handled by the liver, this means that most anticonvulsants will make the pill be broken down more rapidly by the liver, which makes it less effective.

Most of the commonly prescribed oral contraceptives are low-dose pills. **When taken with anticonvulsants, the 'low-dose' pill becomes almost a 'no-dose' pill, with an increased risk of pregnancy.** It is thus important that women taking anticonvulsants should take a high-dose pill, which because of the effect of the anticonvulsants will be reduced to the equivalent of a low-dose pill, but will produce reasonable protection against pregnancy. This is a matter that you should discuss with your doctor. High-dose pills may produce spotting, again something you should discuss with your doctor.

It is also worth mentioning that occasionally some women will find that taking the pill may alter their seizure control either for the better or worse. Should this occur, you should again discuss it with your doctor.

Can you explain the relationship between seizures and menstruation?

The relationship is known as 'catamenial epilepsy' which means seizures either in association with menstruation or made worse by menstruation. How common this relationship is seems uncertain. It would appear that for most women it is not a problem but for some there is a clear relationship. So much so that they can expect a marked deterioration in seizure control either premenstrually or in association with the period itself.

There have been a few studies which have looked at this problem, but have not really provided any very useful answers. There are a number of hormonal changes which take place in association with menstruation but there is not a clear relationship between blood hormone levels and seizures. In addition, it has been shown, at least for phenytoin, that blood levels may fall during a period and this may also contribute. The other theory is that because of fluid retention associated with menstruation, there may be some brain swelling which may make seizures worse.

As the basic cause of the problem is not understood, it is not surprising that management consists of a number of approaches. The two most commonly employed are the use of a diuretic (water tablet) to reduce fluid retention. This may work occasionally but has not been formally studied. More recently it has been shown that the use of clobazam for about 3 days before the period starts and during the period, in other words for about 10 days per month, **may** markedly reduce catamenial epilepsy.

Is medication safe during pregnancy?

This is always a major concern for parents. It is known that there is a slightly higher rate of abnormal babies born to mothers with epilepsy who are taking anticonvulsants when compared to the remainder of the population. Physical abnormalities in the baby have been described with all the commonly used anticonvulsants, with the least abnormalities being described to date with carbamazepine. Babies born to mothers taking carbamazepine may have a smaller head circumference than other babies; however on follow-up to 5 years of age this has not been shown to be any handicap to the children.

The risk of abnormalities in the baby is difficult to assess, but it seems to be commoner in mothers who are taking 3 or more anticonvulsant medications. Bearing in mind that there is anyway about a 2% risk of having a baby with an abnormality in the non-epileptic population, the risk for a mother with epilepsy is probably about 4 per cent. **That is a 96% chance of having a normal baby.**

Does medication need to be changed during pregnancy?

Medication dosage may well need to be altered during pregnancy. Due to the increase in body weight associated with pregnancy and the associated hormonal changes, anticonvulsant blood levels quite often fall. These need to be checked from time to time and the dosage altered if necessary. It is important to remember to reduce the dose after the pregnancy is over.

There may be changes in seizure frequency during pregnancy. Various studies have produced different results in this regard, but as a generalization it might be said that for about 50% of pregnant epileptic women there is no change in seizure frequency, whilst about 25% will either show a deterioration in seizure control or, interestingly, a marked improvement in seizure control. So it is only a relatively small number of women whose seizure control deteriorates during pregnancy.

Finally it is worth mentioning that there is a condition called 'gestational epilepsy' which implies having seizures only when pregnant.

Can you breast feed whilst taking anticonvulsant medication?

Yes you can and should be encouraged to do so. All the anticonvulsant drugs are excreted in breast milk, but in very small amounts and will not do any harm to the baby. Occasionally, especially with the barbiturates, the baby may be a little drowsy. From a practical point of view, if you are worried about having a seizure whilst breast feeding, feed the baby whilst sitting on the floor, that way you cannot really drop the baby.

Will any children I have get epilepsy? My mother had seizures when she was little and now I have developed epilepsy.

This question again stresses the importance of being specific about the type of epilepsy and not talking about 'epilepsy in general'. Most types of epilepsy are not inherited, but there is a familial tendency in childhood absence epilepsy (petit mal). A few other rare types of epilepsy may be inherited. This is a matter which you should discuss with your doctor. (See page 6.)

Chapter 12
Epilepsy and Learning

The future of a child with epilepsy depends a great deal on the management of the condition during the younger years. The attitude adopted at home and at school is very important. These children need to share the company of other children, go to normal schools and partake in the usual activities. They are normal children with a particular problem which is in fact much less disabling for many of them than, for example, asthma might be. Restrictions are often imposed because of unfounded fears; these need to be discussed and avoided.

Some parents and teachers blame any unusual behaviour, such as outbursts of anger or irritability, on the epilepsy. There is usually no connection between the two unless there are clear indications otherwise. However, there is evidence that in some children learning and behaviour problems do arise in connection with their epilepsy. Those with particular types of epilepsy (especially left-sided temporal lobe epilepsy) are more likely to be affected in this way, and boys more so than girls.

What are the school problems?

Children with epilepsy are variously said to be absent minded, lethargic, sleepy and lacking in concentration. Some anticonvulsant drugs may have adverse effects on the child's schoolwork. Difficulties with reading, inattention of various types, dependency and other kinds of disturbed behaviour may occur. An enlightened teacher may take advantage of a seizure in class to explain to the other students about epilepsy. This is useful for the child with epilepsy and the other students. Many children with epilepsy (about 50%, especially boys) have some sort of school problem which may stop them achieving their academic potential. The reasons for this are not entirely clear, but include the following.

1. The effects of the anticonvulsant drugs. Phenobarbitone and primidone may affect concentration span and attention to some extent. Chronic intoxication with phenytoin may lead to intellectual deterioration. There is little information about the other anticonvulsants.
2. Perceptual problems. The information on the effects of epilepsy on reading skills is that:

- the reading skills of children with generalized epilepsy are similar to those of non-epileptic children;
- children, especially boys, with EEG abnormalities or with focal EEG abnormalities on the left side of the brain, read less well than non-epileptic children;
- reading skills of boys with epilepsy, of whatever type, are not as good as those of epileptic girls;
- long-term phenytoin use is associated with lower reading skills than with other anticonvulsants.

In summary, there may be quite definite learning problems in about half of the children with epilepsy, boys more so than girls. These need to be recognized and dealt with as well as possible at an educational level.

Does anticonvulsant medication affect learning?

Yes it may do. In essence it has been shown that barbiturates, phenytoin and clonazepam in usual doses quite frequently affect memory, visual scanning, auditory tasks, mental and motor speed. In high dosage, sodium valproate may have similar, but less marked, effects. Carbamazepine in high dosage may affect concentration and motor speed.

This information is probably sufficiently important to suggest that phenytoin, the barbiturates and clonazepam should not be used as drugs of first choice in the late 1980s. This is particularly the case in children, but is also applicable to adults. Thus, where possible, carbamazepine, sodium valproate and/or clobazam should be regarded as the anticonvulsants of first choice.

Does epilepsy affect mental ability?

Seizures themselves probably do not affect mental ability although one would have to wonder about this in people who have severe and frequent seizures.

However epilepsy itself may be associated with decreased mental ability in some people. This may be for example because they have had a head injury which has left them with brain damage, epilepsy and associated intellectual problems. In people with 'idiopathic' epilepsy, there may be associated learning problems, difficulties with memory and sometimes behavioural difficulties. These may be associated with the epilepsy itself, especially temporal lobe epilepsy, but may also be related to anticonvulsant medications. It has been shown that the 'older generation' of anticonvulsants such as phenytoin, the barbiturates and clonazepam may have a significant effect on mental functioning including difficulties with learning, cognition and memory. This appears to be less of a problem with the newer drugs such as carbamazepine, sodium valproate and clobazam. It is thus worth discussing with your doctor a possible review of your medication if you are concerned about decreasing mental ability.

My memory is poor. What can I do about it?

It may be that even without epilepsy you would have had a poor memory. On the other hand, it is known that people with epilepsy, especially those with temporal lobe epilepsy, have poorer memories than people without epilepsy. This may be made worse by anticonvulsant medication, especially the older drugs (phenytoin, barbiturates and clonazepam).

Discuss the problem with your doctor. Suggest doing an anticonvulsant blood level to ensure that you are not intoxicated with your medication, discuss changing to the newer anticonvulsants (carbamazepine, sodium valproate or clobazam) and consider seeing a clinical psychologist.

People with memory problems can often be assisted by quite simple means to improve the situation. The use of diaries, note pads and memory cues are invaluable and are underutilized by people with epilepsy.

I don't think teachers understand about epilepsy. They are not interested!

This is a common cry. Spare a thought for the teacher who needs to know about a whole range of conditions which could affect their pupils. Epilepsy, diabetes, asthma, arthritis etc.

The epilepsy movement has long been aware of this problem and over the past 3 years the National Epilepsy Association of Australia and the state associations have targeted teachers with information on epilepsy. In the main, teachers have been receptive and indeed have encouraged the National Epilepsy Association of Australia to compile a teachers manual on epilepsy. This will be available in 1989 and interested readers could purchase a copy from their state association and the New Zealand Epilepsy Association.

Chapter 13
Epilepsy and Lifestyle

A long list of dos and don'ts for people with epilepsy is of little help. Most of the problems can be solved by using a bit of common sense. It is important to bear in mind that some people have mild epilepsy and others severe epilepsy. Obviously the person who has a seizure once a year will approach life differently to someone who has a seizure once a week. The factors that need to be taken into account are:

- the type of seizure;
- the severity of the seizure;
- when the seizures occur;
- the age of the patient.

When epilepsy is diagnosed, people are often shocked and frightened. This may lead to some degree of overprotection, particularly of children. But once the seizures are controlled and appropriate explanation and advice has been given, their confidence should grow and they should be encouraged to lead as normal a life as is possible. There are some practical points worthy of mention.

Swimming A person with epilepsy should never swim alone. Always inform a companion of the condition and explain what to do if a seizure should occur. Avoid scuba diving.

Bathing A number of people with epilepsy have drowned in baths. Never leave an epileptic person alone in the house when they are taking a bath; keep the bathroom door ajar and make sure that the bathwater is reasonably shallow. You could also tie a piece of string to your toe and the bathplug.

Showering The risks of showering are threefold.

- If someone has a tonic–clonic seizure in the shower it may be difficult to get at them.
- They might push an arm or a leg through a glass panel.

Showers should be fitted with the best shatterproof glass. Wire-reinforced glass is in fact weaker than sheet glass. A good alternative is a shower curtain.

• The hot tap may be turned on fully when bumped during a fit, resulting in burns. Ideally, a temperature control device should be fitted to the water system in the shower. A water control fitting that operates from under the shower head is less likely to be knocked during a seizure.

Bicycle riding   A person with epilepsy can ride a bicycle taking the normal precautions that any other cyclist should be taking, such as wearing a helmet. Children who have frequent seizures should ride in a protected environment.

Horse riding   A person with epilepsy who wishes to ride a horse should wear a helmet and ride with others.

Climbing   Climbing is not a sensible hobby for people with epilepsy for obvious reasons.

Machinery   Working with unprotected power saws, presses, etc. should be avoided.

Driving   A further problem is that of driving. Today driving a car is an integral part of everyday living. Not being able to drive can be inconvenient and, of course, can limit job prospects. In Australia, the present legal situation, which is under review, is that a person should have been seizure-free for 2 years to obtain a driving licence. In New Zealand the law is that one has to have been seizure free for a year, with no change in medication during that time. Consult your local motor transport office.

Is good nutrition important for good seizure control?

Good nutrition is important for all of us and people with epilepsy are no different in this regard. There is no good evidence that various nutrients, or the lack of them, has any significant effect on seizure control. There has been some work done on trace metals in epilepsy and most of the results are inconclusive. To date there is no evidence that taking trace metals will improve seizure control. Very rarely patients taking sodium valproate may become zinc deficient. This is always associated with a skin rash and responds to zinc supplementation.

It has been known for many years that people taking barbiturates and/or phenytoin may become deficient in folic acid which in turn may lead to anaemia. This, if it occurs at all, is usually seen after these medications have been taken for over 10 years. If anaemia is present, folic acid supplements should be taken. Occasionally, for reasons that are not understood, folic acid supplementation may be associated with a deterioration in seizure control.

Is it possible to get insurance if you have epilepsy?

People with epilepsy seem to have most difficulty in obtaining various types of life insurance. This varies from one insurance company to another. The National Epilepsy Association of Australia has made arrangements specifically for people with epilepsy with an insurance company. Ask your local epilepsy association about this.

Is it safe to drink alcohol?

Opinions differ on this question, but a middle of the road view would be 'Yes, you can have the occasional drink'. Why should people with epilepsy drink very little alcohol? There are probably 3 main reasons. Firstly, alcohol is a depressant and will alter the seizure threshold and may induce seizures. Secondly, because alcohol is a depressant, it will compound any drowsiness associated with your medication and thirdly because it may alter the way in which the anticonvulsant medication is handled in your body.

Finally, do not drink and drive! This is appropriate advice for all of us, but for those with epilepsy who do drive and are taking medication, this is quite definitely a no no.

Can a person with epilepsy take part in sports?

People with epilepsy should be able to do whatever they wish. A commonsense approach is required. For example, a child who has seizures at night only or has two seizures a year will obviously be able to do a lot more than a child who has half a dozen seizures a week. Certain activities such as rock climbing are simply not sensible and people with epilepsy should never swim alone. They should always be with someone who knows that they have epilepsy. Children can ride bicycles observing the same precautions as any other cyclist. In addition there is no reason why people with epilepsy cannot partake in contact sports if they so wish. Seizures are less likely to occur while you are happy doing something requiring your concentration, rather than being bored at home.

Do people with epilepsy need more sleep than normal?

This question is asked because a marked lack of sleep lowers the seizure threshold and may lead to an exacerbation of seizures (see page 81). This is best avoided by having a reasonably regular sleep pattern, but not necessarily having more sleep than anyone else.

A good example of seizures due to sleep deprivation is the story related by a 16-year-old girl who said that she had had 3 seizures over two months; all on Saturday mornings at about midday. On closer questioning, she always went out on Friday nights but on these 3 occasions had only got to bed at about 6 a.m. In addition she had had rather a lot of alcohol. On waking after about 4 or 5 hours sleep, she would have a seizure. It could, and should, be argued that this young woman does not have epilepsy but has had 3 provoked seizures; in her case provoked by a lack of sleep and alcohol, both factors which can reasonably be dealt with.

Should children with epilepsy be treated differently from other children?

The general answer must be no. However it is known that the parents of epileptic children are more overprotective than, for example, the parents of children with asthma or diabetes, let alone children with no health problems. Ideally children with epilepsy should be treated like all other children and should take part in all the activities that other children do, to ensure normal social development. This is however, for some parents, easier said than done.

The unpredictability of seizures at odd times in odd places is a constant worry for parents. Seizure frequency is also an important factor. The child who has 1 seizure every 6 months is obviously going to be able to do more, and be allowed to do more, than a child who has 4 seizures a day. Factors such as the nature of the seizure, seizure frequency and duration and presence or absence of physical/intellectual retardation all impinge on the decision as to how much a child can do. Having said this, as liberal an attitude as possible is to be encouraged.

Do preservatives and colourings affect children with epilepsy?

There is no proven evidence that they do. Even less so than, for example, implicating these substances in asthma or hyperactivity, where it is possible that they play a role. This leads to the question of dietary manipulation in children with epilepsy. There is no evidence that altering the diet has any effect on seizure control with the very rare exception of those young children who may respond to a ketogenic diet. The ketogenic diet, which is quite unpalatable, acts by increasing the blood concentration of a variety of acids in the body which, it is suggested, results in some chemical changes in the brain. Occasionally this may be of help in a child with infantile spasms or myoclonic epilepsy.

Does my blood sugar level affect my seizure pattern?

This question has perhaps two answers. Firstly, seizures may be caused by hypoglycaemia (low blood sugar). This occurs mainly in the newborn period. The hypoglycaemia is usually easily treated, the seizures stop and epilepsy does not ensue. Rarely in the newborn period and in later life, there may be some benign tumours of the pancreas which produce recurrent and unremitting hypoglycaemia. If not diagnosed the recurrent hypoglycaemia may produce brain damage and subsequent epilepsy. The blood sugar should always be tested when a person presents with their first seizure.

The second part of the question raises the issue of the 'presently fashionable' phenomenon of hypoglycaemia. Lay periodicals, magazines and so on are littered with articles about hypoglycaemia, the suggestion being that those who feel listless, out of sorts, weary, depressed etc. are probably hypoglycaemic. Numerous remedies are suggested for this non-existent phenomenon. Blood sugar fluctuates across the day, being highest after meals. Under normal circumstances however, it does not fall into the hypoglycaemic range unless there is a good reason. Ordinary fluctuations in the blood sugar level do not affect seizure frequency. True hypoglycaemia certainly may.

Does epilepsy or do anticonvulsants affect sexuality?

Sexual desire may be reduced in some people with epilepsy for reasons that are not understood. Whether this is due to the epilepsy itself or for psychological reasons is not clear. Very occasionally anticonvulsant medication may contribute to this problem; this is probably due to an effect of the drugs on the sex hormones. This is a matter which should be discussed with your specialist. Overall, the vast majority of people with epilepsy should be able to have a perfectly normal sex life. It is extremely rare that sexual intercourse will bring on a seizure and there is no truth in the myth that too much sex causes epilepsy.

Does a father's epilepsy affect the fertility of his sperm?

There is no evidence that this is the case, nor is there any good evidence that anticonvulsant medications affect male fertility.

Can someone with epilepsy get a driving licence?

Yes they can. The regulations vary from country to country and in Australia from state to state. You should therefore get information from your local motor transport department or epilepsy association. Having said this, the general rule is best summarized by saying that in Australia it should be possible to obtain a driving licence if you have been seizure free for a period of 2 years. There are a number of variations on this general theme, but you would need to inquire locally about those. In New Zealand, the restriction is for a period of 1 year.

I always have an aura before my fits. Can I drive?

If you are still having the fits, with or without auras, you should not be driving. It may be that your aura is in fact sufficiently long for you to pull off the road and avoid an accident; however it would be quite a risk for a doctor to recommend driving on those grounds.

Can I still play sport now that I have epilepsy?

The answer is yes, but must be interpreted in a commonsense way. For someone whose fits are well controlled, there should be no limitation on sporting activity. People with epilepsy should never swim alone and it is wise not to be involved in potentially dangerous pastimes such as rock climbing, climbing tall trees etc. Otherwise all sports and activities should be allowed and encouraged. On the other hand, for the child who has several fits a day, there will obviously be certain logical limitations. This is a matter which should be looked at in a commonsense way and discussed with your doctor or local epilepsy association.

Why did it happen to me?

For many people with epilepsy this is unanswerable. In some people there may be a good reason for their epilepsy such as a difficult birth, meningitis, a head injury, a stroke and so on. However, for most people there is probably a chemical abnormality in their brain, which is only now beginning to be understood. When it is better understood, it should be possible to target the abnormality with more specific medications.

The question 'why me' is a common one and usually arises soon after the shock of being diagnosed as having epilepsy (see Fig. 4). This is part of a grief reaction at having 'lost one's health'. It is a normal question, but as already mentioned, often

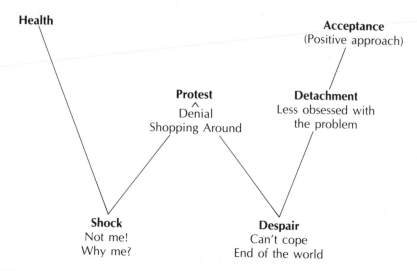

Figure 4. *A diagramatic representation of a grief reaction which occurs when someone dies, or 'loses their health', i.e. develops an illness such as epilepsy. Readers will almost certainly recognize some of the stages that they have been through or may presently be in.*

cannot be answered. It is part of a process which people have to work through to gain acceptance of their condition.

Contrary to common belief, acceptance does not imply defeat. Acceptance means accepting your epilepsy as part and parcel of you as a person. Once you have achieved this, you will feel that you have at least some control over your epilepsy and your life. The importance of 'acceptance' should not be underestimated; it is absolutely crucial in coming to grips with epilepsy. Acceptance is necessary for the person with epilepsy and the entire family.

I am really scared to go out because I can't tell when I am going to have a seizure. What kinds of warning signals might I expect?

It depends on what seizure type you have as to whether you are likely to have a warning (aura) or not. In fact, most people with epilepsy do not have a warning prior to their seizure. Some people, especially with temporal lobe epilepsy, may have an aura. It is generally believed that this is not a seizure, but something which precedes it. This is probably incorrect and it is now felt that **an aura is itself a seizure, probably a partial seizure.** This may then be followed by a complex partial seizure or a tonic–clonic seizure.

You cannot really expect a warning to help you. Epilepsy is an unpredictable condition and it is this unpredictability that people with epilepsy have, with time, to get used to. You need to work towards an understanding and acceptance of your epilepsy, rather than living in hope of having a useful warning.

How do I stop people fussing over me?

Sometimes with difficulty. This is especially a problem for children. It is known that children with epilepsy are more overprotected than children with other chronic illnesses. This is related to the unpredictability of seizures, the fact that parents are often worried that their child may die during a seizure and that they may injure themselves. This 'fussing' is often a sign that the person/people doing it need to work more towards understanding and acceptance.

It takes time for relatives to adapt to a family member having epilepsy and this takes us again to the issue of 'acceptance' (see pages 75–6). Some people never adapt, but with time, most do. It has to be recognized that people with epilepsy are 'normal' the vast majority of the time and have sporadic seizures. Obviously someone who has drop attacks every day needs to be more protected than someone who has a seizure every few months. The degree of protection and fussing should be commonsense, rather than an emotional decision. Easier said than done!

How can I make people realize what it is like to be limited (on occasions)?

Perhaps epilepsy, or any other chronic condition, sorts out friends from acquaintances. You need to be quite up front and clear with people. Know your own epilepsy well, so that you can answer people's questions clearly and with facts, rather than responding emotionally. You should be able to say, for example: 'I have temporal lobe epilepsy which means I have episodes of confusion and wandering about which occur once in a while. I take medication for this'. Further, 'because of the epilepsy there are some things which it is unwise for me to do. I can't drive a car, I don't swim alone, I take very little alcohol'. Your true friends are almost certain to understand, be appreciative that you have explained and confided in them and will support you. Less good friends may be less supportive.

Why can't I have my licence back?

Driving a car implies a responsibility to the passengers in the car and to other road users. You may feel OK to drive, but as seizures are usually unpredictable in their occurrence, you may not be as safe as you think. It is for this reason that there is the very general rule that to drive you should have been seizure free for 2 years (see page 70).

Should I tell people about my epilepsy?

The answer should be yes! The term 'should' is used rather than 'must', as some people find it very difficult to do so because of the stigma of epilepsy. Whilst the stigma should not exist, it does. For example, for someone who has the occasional nocturnal seizure, why tell anyone? Others worry that if they declare their epilepsy, they may not get a job etc. In other words, situations vary greatly.

Ideally, you should declare your epilepsy so that people know about it, about you and how to help you if you have a seizure. Moreover, unless people with epilepsy stand up to be counted, the stigma will persist. It is very much a Catch 22 situation. Certainly if you might endanger yourself or others, it is your clear moral responsibility to declare your epilepsy. Find out the facts first, so that you can present yourself well.

My family treat me like a leper. What can I do about it?

Get help! Discuss the problem with your doctor or local epilepsy association.

Ask them if they would discuss the situation with your family. It is highly likely that they are afraid and do not understand about epilepsy and its implications. Basically they need to be educated and you are probably too close to the whole situation to be able to do anything about it. Getting help from a third party, outside the family, should go some way to resolving the problem. There are many myths which still exist about epilepsy and until people can discuss these and get the facts, they may treat you inappropriately.

I'm scared of my own child because I hate seeing him have a convulsion. How can I overcome this?

Only by discussing it with your doctor, local epilepsy association or someone who has epilepsy. Your reaction is not uncommon and it is something which you have to work through. The reality of the situation is that as things are you are of little help to your son. It takes us back again to the 'acceptance' issue (see pages 75–6). You need to discuss your fears and eventually be reassured that they are in fact irrational. If your son is going to continue to have seizures, then it is vital that you be in a positive frame of mind so as to help him as much as possible.

How can you say personal stress is not the cause of my epilepsy?

There is without doubt a relationship between stress and seizures. This is certainly applicable to stress making seizures more frequent. This is a common event occurring in all age groups and should be managed by recognizing the relationship and trying to deal with the stress rather than taking more and more medication.

What is much less clear is whether stress actually 'starts epilepsy off'. All those involved in the care of people with epilepsy know of anecdotal stories of people who had a stressful or highly emotional experience and sometime thereafter had a seizure. There is however no proof that there is a relationship between the two.

I have noticed that many people with epilepsy appear to have bouts of bronchitis. Is there any connection?

There is almost certainly no connection. Phenytoin and sodium valproate may occasionally alter some aspects of the body's immune system, at least as measured in the blood. These changes however have not been shown to be associated with an actual increase in infections.

Some young children, if handicapped and immobile, especially if they are receiving benzodiazepines (clonazepam, nitrazepam and clobazam) may be recurrently chesty. This is because these agents increase salivation and secretion of mucus in the lungs. In an immobile handicapped child, this accumulates and may lead to recurrent infections.

Chapter 14
Seizure Provoking Factors

There are a number of **provoking factors** which may bring out fits in people with epilepsy. **These are important as they should obviously be avoided if at all possible.** They include:

Lack of sleep

Sleep deprivation is known to alter the electrical activity of the brain and thus may provoke seizures. This is particularly the case in young adults who like to stay up late at night, but is important for epileptics of all ages. A good night's sleep is strongly recommended, albeit that a 'good night's sleep' is a very individual thing. Some people need more sleep than others.

Menstruation

It has long been recognized that women may have a deterioration in seizure control either just before, or in association with, their periods. The cause of this phenomenon, which is called catamenial epilepsy, is not understood although it may relate to the retention of fluid, possible alterations in hormonal balance, or changes in the blood levels of anticonvulsants which sometimes occur in association with menstruation.

Stress

This is a very difficult area, as what is stressful for one person may not be for someone else. It is important for people whose seizures are made worse by stress to appreciate this, as no amount of anticonvulsant medication will solve the problem. Often more and more medication is given, leading to quite severe side effects such as drowsiness, unsteadiness and some degree of confusion.

Alcohol

This is often combined with a lack of sleep. Alcohol acts by removing inhibiting factors, as you can observe by watching anyone who has had too much to drink. It is this lack of inhibition of brain cells which probably accounts for the fits which may occur with alcohol. The seizures usually occur in the hangover (morning after) period. People with epilepsy should drink very modestly indeed, both for this reason and also because it may interfere with some anticonvulsant medications. Alcoholics who suddenly stop drinking may have withdrawal seizures; these seizures, however, do not represent epilepsy.

Infections

This applies especially in childhood. It is common to observe that, when a child whose seizures are normally well-controlled develops an infection such as tonsillitis, the seizures go out of control. This is probably related to the fever that is associated with the infection and the deterioration usually lasts 2 to 4 days. **It is particularly important for parents to be aware of this association as it makes coping with the situation much easier.**

Drugs

Some drugs may precipitate convulsions. These include the tricyclic antidepressants, phenothiazines and very high doses of penicillin. The withdrawal of drugs, such as barbiturates and Valium, may also cause seizures. None of the illegal, street drugs is in any way recommended in those with epilepsy.

Is there a relationship between puberty and the start of epilepsy?

This is a slightly vexed question as there is not an absolute answer. It has become enshrined in some books there is a relationship between puberty and epilepsy. It is said that epilepsy may commence in association with puberty or that seizures may get worse at this time. There is no doubt that a few people have their first seizure around about puberty and may subsequently go on to develop epilepsy. This does not necessarily mean that puberty was causative. There is no proof of the relationship between the two.

On the other hand, most doctors involved in the care of children with epilepsy will have encountered some children, especially girls, in whom seizure control does appear to deteriorate in association with puberty. The reason for this is unclear and as for catamenial epilepsy, there may be a hormonal cause (see page 81). There appears to be little that can be done about this sort of seizure exacerbation, which usually lasts for months to about a year and then settles back to the previous seizure pattern.

Can anything trigger off fits?

Yes there are a number of things which can stimulate (provoke, trigger) seizures. Essentially they all work by lowering the seizure threshold which is a balance between the negative (inhibitory) and positive (excitatory) influence which are brought to bear on the brain cells. It is this balance which prevents seizures from occurring. When it is disturbed, i.e. when the seizure threshold is lowered, seizures may occur.

The factors which lower the seizure threshold include intercurrent illness especially with fever, fever itself, alcohol, lack of sleep, stress and menstruation. Any of these factors may be associated with an increase in seizure frequency. It is important if seizures are provoked in this manner that attention be paid to the provoking factor and its avoidance, rather than just increasing the dosage of regular medication.

Will jet lag affect my epilepsy?

It is difficult to think that jet lag would affect seizure control other than by association with fatigue (see page 81). If you were to miss an entire night's sleep, you may become tired enough for a seizure to be provoked, but even that is not terribly likely.

Will discipline bring on a seizure in a child?

Whilst this might occasionally occur, it would be very uncommon indeed. It is important to bear in mind in young children that breath-holding attacks may occur, look very much like seizures and are frequently associated with discipline, being thwarted etc. As has already been discussed (page 81), stress may be associated with an increase in seizure frequency. In this regard, although discipline might be regarded as a stress, it is very uncommon for it to provoke seizures.

It is important that children with epilepsy be treated as would be other children and not overprotected, spoilt and cossetted. It is known that children with epilepsy are more over-protected and dependent than, for example, children with asthma or diabetes, let alone children who have no illness to cope with. There is, as with all children, a need for firm, sensible discipline.

Chapter 15
Getting a Job

Employment may present problems for people with epilepsy. Obviously some occupations are just not suitable for people with epilepsy; driving a bus, working with heavy or dangerous machinery or working on a scaffold would not be sensible. Two factors need to be taken into account: the possibility that those with epilepsy may injure themselves during a seizure or that they may cause harm to others.

What occupations are closed to those with epilepsy? The armed forces will not employ someone with epilepsy. Other examples include occupations such as an airline pilot, public transport driver, crane driver, etc. It is logical and appropriate that people with epilepsy should not be involved in these occupations.

More of a problem is the **prejudice** against persons with epilepsy. This leads to the perennial problem of whether people should declare their epilepsy or try to hide it. Ideally it is best to declare your epilepsy and hope that the prospective employer will understand. Sadly this is not always the case. This is a real problem and is likely to persist. It is hoped that through the efforts of national epilepsy associations and the various state organisations throughout the world, this problem will lessen with the passage of time as public awareness increases. Unfortunately there is no easy solution to this very real problem.

Should I declare my epilepsy when going for a job?

The correct answer to this has to be yes. However it also has to be accepted that some people with epilepsy are still discriminated against, especially with regard to prospective employment. This leads to a 'chicken and egg situation'. Which comes first? If you say you have epilepsy, you may not get the job. If you don't declare it and have a seizure, you may well be fired. The stress of not declaring your epilepsy may also precipitate seizures.

On balance it is better to declare one's epilepsy, be prepared to discuss it, face the prejudice and work towards minimizing it, rather than hide the condition. **It is after all only by people with epilepsy 'coming out of the closet' and being counted, that things for epileptics will in fact improve in society at large. It is thus the responsibility of people with epilepsy to help themselves and this is one way of doing it.**

What type of job can I get?

Almost any kind of job is open to you. There are certain restrictions for those with epilepsy which are designed to protect them and society at large. In other words, the restricted jobs are those where the risk of having a seizure would be unacceptable in terms of safety. Such jobs include the armed forces, the police force, driving public transport vehicles, airline pilots etc. You would agree that it would be unwise for people with epilepsy to hold such occupations.

Over and above these genuine restrictions there is a general feeling that it is more difficult to get a job if you have epilepsy. This may well be true and often leads people to conceal their epilepsy. There is without doubt some degree of discrimination against people with epilepsy, but this is probably not as frequent as folklore would suggest. So any job is open to you, but you must weigh up the risks.

My seizures have recently become more frequent. Should I change my occupation?

The need to look for another job should be a secondary issue. If you are worried about your job because of a recent deterioration in seizure control, it would be most logical to ask why the seizures have got worse. This should be looked at first, rather than changing jobs.

The seizures may have become worse for one, or a combination, or reasons. It may be that your epilepsy has changed, that there is a need for a review of your medication or that some outside factor such as stress is altering your seizure frequency.

The starting point should be to look at the epilepsy rather than changing jobs.

Can I be dismissed from my job if I am seizure free?

The question really should read 'Can I be dismissed from my job simply because I have epilepsy, although I am symptom free'. The answer to this must be no, although this does occur from time to time. If confronted by this situation, it would be important to discuss the matter with your local epilepsy association, the Human Rights Commission and in addition possibly seek legal advice.

Chapter 16
Outlook for People with Epilepsy

From a practical point of view, epilepsy can be divided into 4 categories of severity (see Table 3). Most people with epilepsy fall into the 'significant' epilepsy group.

Overall the outlook for most people with epilepsy is good in terms of seizure control and possible remission of symptoms. For example, about 50% of children with generalized seizures (absence epilepsy and tonic–clonic epilepsy) will be seizure free in adolescence. About 95% of children with benign focal epilepsy of childhood will also become seizure free. In addition many people with photosensitive epilepsy will become seizure free in the third or fourth decade of life.

It is hoped that the situation will improve further with the advent of new medications.

Do you grow out of epilepsy?

With the exception of a particular type of epilepsy seen in childhood called 'benign focal epilepsy of childhood' which ceases at, or around, puberty, most people do not 'grow out of' epilepsy. This does not mean, however, that for many people epilepsy cannot be controlled and that they may come off medication and be seizure free.

In simple terms it can be said that for those who have a brain abnormality, such as that resulting from a birth injury, meningitis or a head injury, the chances of obtaining total seizure control and coming off treatment are not as good as for those in whom there is no obvious cause for their epilepsy. Whilst it is difficult to give accurate figures on the outlook for different types of epilepsy, certain generalizations can be made which should be interpreted in discussion with your doctor.

- Childhood absence epilepsy (Petit Mal): about 50% to 60% of children with this form of epilepsy will be seizure free and

Trivial epilepsy

Few attacks
To treat or not?
Motivation to take medication?
Recurrence/deterioration

Significant epilepsy (The majority of epileptics)

Established diagnosis
Treatment essential
Social stigma
Psychological problems

Disabling epilepsy

Severe/frequent attacks
Physical/intellectual problems
Social decompensation
Compliance problems

Life-destroying epilepsy

Uncontrollable
Continuing care – ?institution
Wasteful of human resources

Table 3. *A practical classification of epilepsy. (Modified from Dr Andrew Black of Adelaide.)*

able to come off medication around about adolescence. The remainder, especially those who have childhood absences and other seizure types (usually tonic–clonic seizures) are likely to carry their epilepsy through into adult life.

- Tonic–clonic (Grand Mal) seizures: this is probably the type of seizure which responds best to treatment and in which it might be expected that 50% to 60% of people will be able to come off treatment and be seizure free.
- Complex partial seizures (temporal lobe epilepsy): in this type of epilepsy it is known from experience that the response to treatment is often rather poor and the chances of being totally seizure free and coming off medication is slight.

As a generalization, the longer it has taken to control the seizures, the more medications required and the more severe the epilepsy, the less likely it is that the person will 'grow out of' their epilepsy. Certain types of epilepsy which occur in young children such as infantile spasms or the Lennox-Gastaut syndrome are known to have a particularly bad outlook for seizure control and are almost always associated with mental retardation.

What is acceptable seizure control?

This is a question so often asked by people with epilepsy and health professionals. There is no absolute answer in terms of the number of seizures per day/week/month or year.

If it is accepted that **treatment is a balance between seizure control and drug side effects** and it is accepted that the epileptic person is best informed about both of these, then it must follow that it is the person with epilepsy who must decide for themselves what 'acceptable seizure control' is. This will vary depending upon the nature of the person concerned, the type of seizures, their frequency, the timing of their occurrence, age, occupation, drug side effects and so on.

'Ideal' seizure control would be to have no seizures at all. This however may not be achievable for some people and for others may only be achieved at a considerable cost in drug side effects. In the latter case it may not be acceptable to that individual. So in a practical world 'acceptable seizure control' is that which is acceptable to the individual with epilepsy. This is an end point which should be reached after mature discussion with your doctor and others who may be involved in your treatment.

This concept does not mean that you should not be aiming at the best seizure control possible, but simply suggests that this may fall short of eradicating seizures totally and also takes into account the matter of drug side effects.

Should all fits go away with medication?

The answer to this question is that this may be what you would like to have happen, but it may well not occur.

It is suggested that going onto anticonvulsant treatment means that most people taking anticonvulsants will have less seizures than before treatment and for some people it may mean the complete eradication of the seizures. In other words **it does not mean that going onto treatment necessarily means that you will never have another fit,** it simply means that you are likely to have less fits. If you are fortunate you may not have any more.

Treatment then is a balance between on the one hand seizure control and on the other drug side effects. It is vital to remember that it is you, the person with epilepsy, that has both the seizures and may have the drug side effects. **This means that you are the best informed person with regard to *your* epilepsy.** Do not forget this. If you appreciate this fact, it should allow you to feel that, within reason, you have the power to have some influence over your own epilepsy.

What does adapting to, and accepting, epilepsy mean?

With any chronic problem, over the passage of time one gets used to it and may actually accept it. The concept of 'acceptance' in coming to grips with a condition like epilepsy is very important. In fact, it might be fair to say that without acceptance, that person never really comes to grips with their problem (see pages 75–6).

When someone is told that they have an illness such as diabetes, heart disease or epilepsy they are shocked. They have moved from good health to illness. In the case of epilepsy, because of the social stigma, this may be even more of a shock. For some people it is like a death sentence. Many people go through a process similar to grieving and begin to ask questions (see Figure 4). They may go through a number of phases such as shock; why me? What have I done to deserve this? Why not the guy next door? This may be followed by a stage of protest where the person will deny having the problems or may go 'shopping around' for various opinions. A second opinion is often very desirable, but seeing doctor after doctor whilst denying reality is of little help. This may be followed by a phase of despair as if the end of the world is at hand where the person just cannot cope. This will usually be followed by a stage of detachment where they are able to stand back from the situation and realize that life is continuing and with luck this will lead to the pinnacle of success, acceptance. Not everyone goes through all these stages, nor do they necessarily go through them in that order; however most people go through some of them. Some get stuck along the way and then go forwards, others get stuck permanently.

Why is acceptance so important? This is because without acceptance your epilepsy will never become part of you and thus you will never come to grips with it and feel that you have any control over it. There is a misconception that acceptance means defeat. Quite the reverse is true; acceptance means accepting that your epilepsy is a part of you in the same way that you might have red hair, blue eyes, a long nose or be tall. You may not like any of the attributes but you are after all stuck with them and the sooner you accept them and get on with living, the better.

Those with epilepsy who do not accept it are often obsessed with their condition and thus let it rule their lives. This is most undesirable. As part of one's clinical practice there is little more gratifying than seeing acceptance dawn on someone with epilepsy; it quite revolutionizes their lives.

Can you stop taking medication after the fits have stopped?

Yes indeed you can. The general approach to this is that if someone has been seizure free for 1 to 4 years (on average 2 years) then it is appropriate to consider coming off medication. The slower this is done, the more likely it is to be successful. Some people will not wish to come off treatment as they feel secure taking their medication; others may see this quite differently.

However you approach this matter, the reality is that the only way in which you will know if you are going to be seizure free when you are off medication is to try and see what happens. It is this risk that some people are not willing to take. There are no tests which will accurately predict if you will be seizure free after coming off medication.

What can be reasonably accurately predicted is that if your seizures have been very difficult to control or there is evidence of brain damage and thus a permanent brain abnormality, then the chances of relapsing are much higher if you come off medication than if those factors did not exist. But even then, some people with these two adverse factors will come off treatment and be seizure free.

There is thus no black and white answer to this problem, which makes the decision to come off medication rather more difficult for the patient to make.

Can a person die during a seizure?

Yes, people may die during a seizure. Fortunately this occurs very rarely indeed.

Very occasionally someone may die during, or as a result of, status epilepticus. This presumably is because the seizure(s) have lasted for a very long time and as a result there has been inadequate oxygen taken into the body which may affect the heart and brain. Other causes of death during a seizure include: drowning if a seizure occurs in water or if a seizure occurs in a particularly dangerous place leading to a fatal injury.

Can epilepsy injure the brain?

This is a difficult question to answer accurately as 'epilepsy' cannot, and should not, be generalized about. Epilepsy occurs in different types and different degrees of severity. In other words, epilepsy is not a uniform condition. In severe, tonic–clonic seizures which are prolonged and may last for hours, often associated with poor breathing which leads to an inadequate amount of oxygen in the blood (hypoxia), there may be some brain damage. These prolonged seizures or seizures which occur one after the other for a long time are called status epilepticus and represent a medical emergency. Help should be sought from your doctor, ambulance service or local hospital to bring the seizures to an end.

It has become common practice, especially with children who have difficult epilepsy, for parents to have Valium at home to be administered rectally. This has been shown to be very effective in controlling, or at least lessening, status epilepticus. This practice is acceptable to most parents and is to be commended. You may wish to discuss this with your doctor.

Can epilepsy be cured?

In general, when talking of epilepsy, one does not speak of 'cure' but 'remission'. This means that the seizures have ceased and the person may be off all medication. Remission may last indefinitely and thus may be the equivalent of a cure. However there is a possibility, however remote, that a seizure may recur if provoked by factors such as fever, alcohol, a marked lack of sleep etc. This is because these factors lower the 'seizure threshold' and make seizures, in those predisposed to them, more likely. It is thus perhaps wise never to say to patients 'you will never again have a seizure', as this cannot be absolutely guaranteed.

The exception to this general rule is a condition called benign focal epilepsy of childhood in which seizures are known to cease at puberty or shortly thereafter. Once the seizures have ceased they do not recur and thus the child can be regarded as cured.

Does epilepsy get worse with age?

For people who have established epilepsy, there is no specific deterioration with age. For those who develop epilepsy in later life, especially in middle or old age, it is more likely than earlier in life that there is an underlying brain abnormality such as a tumour, blood vessel abnormality, stroke etc. These underlying problems may make the epilepsy more difficult to control.

Will frequent seizures cause me to suffer brain damage? My sister is mentally retarded and I've been told I've got epilepsy. Will I go mad too?

Firstly being mentally retarded does not imply being mad. It may imply being slow, perhaps behaving a little strangely from time to time, but it does not imply madness. Nor is there any established relationship between epilepsy and madness. On the other hand, there are some forms of epilepsy which occur in early childhood (infantile spasms and the Lennox-Gastaut syndrome) which are usually associated with mental retardation.

The present evidence is that the occasional seizure is harmless from the point of view of mentation. However frequent, severe, prolonged seizures or recurrent bouts of status epilepticus may cause brain damage, which may affect intellectual development. This emphasizes the need for good seizure control.

Is migraine connected to epilepsy?

This is a very difficult area for there is a relationship between the two, but it is unclear and complicated. There are certainly some people, albeit few, in whom the two conditions co-exist. As the basic problem in migraine is an alteration in blood vessel tone, it may be that this can also affect blood vessels reaching the brain cortex, that part of the brain from which seizures arise. In some people in whom there is a relationship between epilepsy and migraine, both symptoms will improve with anticonvulsant therapy. In other people, there may be a need for anticonvulsant therapy and additional treatment for the migraine.

Will my recently diagnosed 17-year-old son grow out of epilepsy?

This question is included as it exemplifies an important educational point. This is that the question is unanswerable in the way in which it is posed. It lacks specific information on the nature of the boy's epilepsy, the age of onset, the frequency of seizures and so on.

It is therefore useful to use this question to suggest how best to structure a question to obtain the most useful reply. This might be along the following lines.

'My son, aged 17, was diagnosed as having tonic-clonic epilepsy 15 months ago. He is taking carbamazepine 400mg twice daily and since going onto medication has had 3 seizures over a year. Will he grow out of it?'

With this information there is at least a chance that a sensible discussion might take place. **It is very important that people with epilepsy present their predicament clearly and concisely. To do this they need to be well informed in the first place.**

My son has tuberous sclerosis and his seizures seem to be changing. Why? For a while he seems to be OK on his medication and then it doesn't seem to work? What should we do? We have taken him off everything at the moment. Will this make his epilepsy worse?

There is no answer to your question except to say that what you describe can and does occur. The reason for this phenomenon is not clear.

You can really only do one of three things. Increase the dose to see if that helps or if drug intoxication occurs. Change to another anticonvulsant, building up the dose until it is effective and then withdraw the previous drug. The final alternative is to withdraw the medication slowly (over weeks/months) and see what happens. This is what you have done.

It is not possible to predict if this will make him worse or not. You will only know by trying. If as he is coming off the medication the fits become more frequent, then it is highly likely that the drug was having at least some effect and should probably be reintroduced.

Chapter 17
Doctor–Patient Relationship

Epilepsy associations often hear the complaints 'My doctor is not interested', 'My doctor does not know much about epilepsy'. In fact in a number of surveys, the frequency of these complaints are not as common as hearsay would suggest.

There are of course people who have difficulty in communicating with their doctor. There are also times when doctors find patients very trying. In essence, there may be faults on both sides. This is all the more reason for people with epilepsy to be well informed about their condition, so that they can have a sensible conversation with their doctor. Communication is a two-way process.

It is well known that most patients forget at best half of the information given them during a consultation. This means that it is necessary for the doctor to repeat important information several times and for the patient to ask questions until the explanation is clear and understood.

It is often very useful to have a written 'shopping list' of questions so that they are not forgotten. Ask the questions early in the consultation to avoid any risk of not obtaining answers. Always ask questions before your prescription is written out as this traditionally means the consultation is almost over.

Am I allowed to change my doctor? How do I do this?

You do not have to ask permission to be 'allowed' to change your doctor. It is your right to seek another opinion at any time.

If you wish to see another doctor, ask your present doctor to kindly refer you for a second opinion. If he/she refuses, you should insist. Firstly, it is your right to have another opinion and secondly your doctor has no right to refuse to assist you. Should this approach not work, discuss it with your local epilepsy association.

By all means, seek a second opinion, but beware of excessive shopping around. Getting too many opinions may be confusing and counter-productive. You need to find a doctor with whom you are comfortable, who is reasonably well informed about epilepsy or one who is prepared to find out and who is interested in you as a person.

My doctor never asks about the effect of my epilepsy on my life, but always does blood tests.

You need to try to redirect your doctor's attention to discuss the issues which **you feel** are important. If your seizures are well controlled, it is probably not necessary to do blood tests at each visit (see page 46). You are at liberty to decline the blood tests if you so wish. Try to redirect the conversation. If you cannot do this, you may wish to see another doctor. Discuss this with your local epilepsy association.

My doctor is so busy that I feel guilty if I ask questions.

This is a very unsatisfactory situation. If you feel dissatisfied, then something is wrong. If your doctor is that busy, he or she is of little help to you. You need to state clearly that there are issues that you need to discuss; if this is not heeded, perhaps you should seek another opinion.

Somehow or other I never get around to ask the questions that I want to.

Write them down. Go into the consultation with your list and say 'There are a few questions that I would like to ask you' and off you go.

Chapter 18
First Aid for Seizures

The only seizures which really require first aid are tonic–clonic (grand mal) and simple partial (focal) seizures. The first aid rules are shown in figure 5.

Can you swallow your tongue during a seizure?

No, it is not possible to swallow one's tongue during a seizure or at any other time. This is one of the great epileptic myths which relates to the fact that during a major (grand mal, tonic–clonic seizure) people often make a choking, gurgling noise and indeed appear to be choking. This is because the muscles of the throat and chest are involved in the seizure and are functioning in a poorly coordinated way and thus the person cannot swallow properly. This leads to an accumulation of saliva in the mouth which accounts both for the choking noise and the frothing at the mouth which occurs in major seizures.

The practice of trying to insert something in the mouth or prise the jaws apart is pointless and dangerous. It leads to broken teeth and bitten fingers and should be avoided. Simply turn the person onto their side, lift their chin and loosen anything tight around the neck. There is no need to do anything more than this.

Should I wear a bracklet or neck chain indicating that I have epilepsy?

This is often very useful and need not be unsightly. The most useful are probably bracelets which unscrew and contain a slip of paper with information on the type of epilepsy, the medication being taken, your name, address and telephone number and that of your doctor.

What to do if someone has a major fit (Grand Mal Fit)

If the person falls near something dangerous like a fire, move them away; otherwise do not move the patient.

Do not try to force anything between the teeth.

If you force an object between the teeth you will break them or get your fingers bitten. Tongues heal – broken teeth do not!

As soon as the jerking stops and breathing starts, make sure that the patient can breathe freely.

Loosen clothing around the neck and turn the head to the side so that the tongue does not fall back. (It is impossible to swallow one's tongue as it is firmly fixed to the floor of the mouth.)

Do nothing more!! Leave the person to recover.

DO NOT:
- slap the face
- try to 'bring the person round'
- give anything to drink
- restrain unless it is absolutely essential

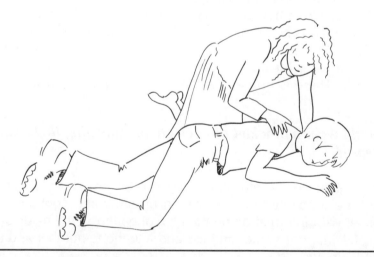

Figure 5. First aid rules.

Should you always call an ambulance when someone has a fit?

There is no clear answer to this question as it depends on the type of seizure, how often the person has seizures, how long they usually last, where they have occurred (e.g. in water) or if they are injured.

Quite obviously if someone with epilepsy has a seizure in a public place when they are alone, passers by will react by calling an ambulance. This may not be necessary and if they had been accompanied by a friend or relative who knew for example that the seizure was likely to be brief, an ambulance would not have been called. In other words, experience in observing and dealing with seizures alters the decision as to when to call for help. It is not uncommon for the parents of children who have just been diagnosed as having epilepsy to call an ambulance for each seizure for the first few seizures. Thereafter, when they realize that the seizures will stop spontaneously after a few minutes, they feel less need to call for help.

The most practical answer to this question is; if you feel the need to call an ambulance when someone is having a seizure, then go ahead and call them. In addition, if the seizure has lasted for 5 minutes or more, help should be sought. Frequently by the time the ambulance arrives, the seizure will have ceased. That does not matter; the presence of the ambulance staff is often very reassuring.

Chapter 19
Drugs Used in the Treatment of Epilepsy

Side effects related to excessive (over) dosage are shown in italic.

Carbamazepine

Carbamazepine is available in 200mg and 100mg tablets as well as a suspension (100mg/5ml). The drug does not last very long in the body and so needs to be taken 2 or 3 times a day.

Side effects with carbamazepine are few but include *sleepiness and double vision*; this usually means that you are taking too much medicine. A rash, like measles, may occur during the first month of treatment. If it does, you are sensitive to the drug and should probably stop taking it after discussion with your doctor.

Patients on carbamazepine should avoid taking the antibiotic erythromycin, as it may make the blood level of carbamazepine rise and produce toxicity. The same applies to Verapamil which is occasionally used in the treatment of epilepsy.

Clobazam

Clobazam is available as a 10mg tablet. It is not a drug that can be used on its own; it needs to be used with another anticonvulsant (adjunct therapy). It can be taken twice daily. Side effects are few, but include some drowsiness, weight gain and, occasionally, depression.

As for clonazepam, tolerance may occur.

Clonazepam

Clonazepam is available in 0.5 and 2.0mg tablets and as a liquid (2.5mg/ml). Clonazepam generally needs to be taken 2 or 3 times a day. Side effects are quite frequent, more so in children than adults. The side effects include hyperactivity, an increase in weight, drowsiness, *slurred speech and an unsteady walk* (as if drunk). There may also be increased salivation.

In some patients, tolerance occurs. This means that they 'get used' to the drug. In these patients, seizures may recur, usually 1 to 6 months after treatment was begun.

Ethosuximide

Ethosuximide is available as a 250mg capsule and a syrup (250mg/5ml).

It lasts a long time in the body and so may be taken once a day although it is usually given twice daily.

Side effects are few and include a decrease in appetite, abdominal pain, tiredness, headache and an *unsteady walk*.

Nitrazepam

Nitrazepam is available as a 5mg tablet and is usually given twice daily. Side effects are similar to those described for clonazepam, but to a lesser extent.

Phenobarbitone

Phenobarbitone is available in 15mg, 30mg, 60mg and 100mg tablets and as a 15-mg/5ml syrup.

Phenobarbitone lasts a long time in the body and can be given once daily although it is usually given twice a day. It has been used for many years as an anticonvulsant, but tends to make patients rather drowsy. Children and elderly people may behave the opposite way and become hyperactive. These behaviour changes have made phenobarbitone less popular now than it was 10 years ago.

Patients on phenobarbitone should not take warfarin (to thin the blood), phenylbutazone (for arthritis), prednisone (for arthritis or asthma) or doxycycline (for infections) without careful medical supervision.

Phenytoin

Phenytoin is available in 30mg capsules, 50mg tablets (chewable), 100mg capsules and 2 suspensions (30mg/5ml and 100mg/5ml).

Phenytoin is retained in the body for a long time and can be used once daily.

It has rather a lot of side effects, although many patients' seizures are well controlled on this drug with minimal side effects. *Drowsiness, double vision, unsteady walk and slurred speech* suggest that the patient has been taking too much of the drug and should contact his/her doctor. Other side effects include swelling of the gums, rashes, acne and an increase in body hair.

Patients on phenytoin should not take rifampicin (for tuberculosis), chloramphenicol (for infections), phenylbutazone (for arthritis), dicoumarol (to thin the blood) or cimetidine (for stomach ulcers) without careful medical supervision.

Primidone

Primidone is available as a 250mg tablet. The drug is broken down to phenobarbitone in the body. (See phenobarbitone).

Sodium valproate

Sodium valproate is available as a 100mg crushable tablet, a 200mg and 500mg enteric-coated tablet, a syrup (200mg/5ml) and a sugar-free liquid (200mg/5ml).

Sodium valproate stays in the body for quite a long time and may be given once daily. It is more usual to give it twice daily.

The side effects of sodium valproate are relatively few and include drowsiness, an increase in weight, hair loss (which is usually temporary) and very rarely jaundice (turning yellow). This last complication (jaundice) is serious and immediate medical attention should be sought. It occurs very rarely and is due to liver damage caused by the drug. If a patient taking this medication feels generally unwell, unduly tired or drowsy and has an increase in seizure frequency, a doctor should be consulted immediately.

Appendix 1
Available Literature

Contact your local epilepsy association (see Appendix 3) for copies of these books.

Books for Children

What difference does it make Danny? by H. Young.
Learning about Epilepsy by R. G. Beran.
I have Epilepsy by Althea.

Books for Parents

Childhood Epilepsy by N. Buchanan.

Books about Epilepsy in General

People with Epilepsy by M.V. and J. Laidlaw.
The Epilepsy Reference Book by P.M. Jeavons and A. Aspinall.
Epilepsy and You by N. Buchanan.
Epilepsy Explained by M.V. and J. Laidlaw.
Epilepsy by P. Hazeldine.

Appendix 2
Trade Names of Commonly Used Anticonvulsant Medications

DRUG	Australia	Britain	Canada	New Zealand	South Africa	United States
Carbamazepine	Tegretol (Geigy) Teril (Alphapharm)	Tegretol (Geigy)	Tegretol (Geigy)	Tegretol (Geigy)	Tegretol (Geigy) Carpaz (Rolab) Degranol (Lennon)	Tegretol (Geigy)
Clobazam	Frisium (Hoechst)	Frisium (Hoechst)		Frisium (Hoechst)	Urbanol (Cassenne/ Roussel)	
Clonazepam	Rivotril (Roche)	Rivotril (Roche)	Rivotril (Roche)	Rivotril (Roche)	Rivotril (Roche)	Clonopin (Roche)
Ethosuximide	Zarontin (Parke Davis)	Zarontin (Parke Davis) Emeside (Lab of Applied Biology)	Zarontin (Parke Davis)	Zarontin (Parke Davis)	Zarontin (Parke Davis)	Zarontin (Parke Davis)
Nitrazepam	Mogadon (Roche) Alodorm (Alphapharm) Dormicum (Protea) Nitepam (USV)	Mogadon (Roche) Nitrados (Berk) Noctased (Unumed) Remnos (DDSA) Somnite (Norgine) Surem (Galen) Unisomnia (Unigreg Vestric)	Mogadon (Roche)	Mogadon (Roche) Insoma 5 (Pacific) Nitepam (USV) Nitraclos (Douglas)	Mogadon (Roche) Arem (Lennon) Lyladorm (MPS Labs) Noctene (Adcock Ingtom) Ormadon (Ormed) Paxadorm (Geo Schwulst) Somnipar (Rolab)	

Phenytoin/ Phenytoin Sodium	Dilantin (Parke Davis)	Epanutin (Parke Davis)	Dilantin (Parke Davis)	Dilantin (Parke Davis)	Epanutin (Parke Davis)	Dilantin (Parke Davis) Diphenylan (Lannett) Pheny Sod. prompt (Zenith/schein/Elkins-Suin)
Primidone	Mysoline (ICI) Midone (Protea)	Mysoline (ICI)	Mysoline (Ayerst)	Mysoline (ICI)	Mysoline (ICI)	Mysoline (Ayerst) Primidone (Danbury/ schein) Myidone Major (Ayerst)
Sodium Valproate	Epilim (Reckitt Colman) Valcote (Abbott)	Epilim (Labaz)	Depakene (Abbott)	Epilim (Reckitt Colman)	Epilim (Labaz)	Depakene (Abbott)

107

Appendix 3

Epilepsy Associations in Australia and New Zealand

Australian Epilepsy Associations

National Epilepsy Association of Australia	PO Box 554, Lilydale Vic. 3140. Telephone: (03) 735 0211.
Australian Capital Territory	Epilepsy Association of the ACT Inc. Shout Office, Hughes Community Centre, Wisdom Street, Hughes ACT 2605. Telephone: (062) 81 2983, 81 2984.
New South Wales	Epilepsy Association of NSW 468 Pennant Hills Road, Pennant Hills NSW 2120. PO Box 521, Pennant Hills NSW 2120. Telephone: (02) 875 1855.
Queensland	Epilepsy Association of Queensland Inc. Room 322, Penney's Building, 210 Queen Street, Brisbane, Qld 4000. Telephone: (07) 229 3606.
South Australia	Epilepsy Association of SA Inc. 471 Regency Road, Prospect SA 5082. PO Box 596, Prospect East SA 5082 Telephone: (08) 269 3511.

Tasmania

Epilepsy Association of Tasmania Inc.
a) 86 Hampden Road, Battery Point,
Hobart Tas. 7000.
PO Box 421,
Sandy Bay Tas. 7005.
Telephone: (002) 34 6967

b) Community Health Centre,
McHugh Street,
Kings Meadow, Launceston Tas. 7249.
(003) 44 5733

Victoria

Epilepsy Foundation of Victoria
818–822 Burke Road,
Camberwell Vic. 3124
Telephone: (03) 813 2866.

Western Australia

West Australian Epilepsy Association
(Inc.)
14 Bagot Road,
Subiaco WA 6008.
Telephone: (09) 381 1187.

New Zealand Epilepsy Associations

Auckland
PO Box 5714,
Auckland.

Telephone: (09) 687 639

Christchurch
PO Box 2468,
Christchurch.

Telephone: (03) 798 175

Far North Interest Group
C/– Matariki Place,
R.D. Tokerau Beach,
Kaitaia.

Telephone: (KTA) 1813J

Hawkes Bay
PO Box 3216,
Onekawa, Napier.

Telephone: (070) 449 766

Manawatu
C/– 12 Glasgow Street,
Palmerston North.

Telephone: (063) 83 769

Nelson
PO Box 2179,
Stoke, Nelson.

Telephone: (054) 68 595

New Zealand Epilepsy Association
PO Box 1074,
Hamilton.

Telephone: (071) 478 472

Otago
PO Box 1142,
Dunedin

Telephone: (024) 771 751

Rotorua Interest Group
PO Box 5059
Rotorua.

Telephone: (073) 84 916

Southland
PO Box 68,
Invercargill.

Telephone: (021) 83 089

Taranaki Interest Group
PO Box 636,
New Plymouth.

Telephone: (067) 88 920

Taupo
PO Box 756,
Taupo.

Telephone: (074) 87 143

Tauranga
PO Box 408,
Tauranga.

Thames Coromandel Interest Group
C/– 671 Pollen Street,
Thames.

Telephone: (0843) 86 375

Thames Valley Interest Group
PO Box 95
Te Aroha.

Telephone: (0819) 48 185

Timaru
PO Box 2060,
Washdyke.

Telephone: (056) 80 574

Tokoroa
PO Box 341,
Tokoroa.

Telephone: (0814) 69 831

Waikato
PO Box 683,
Hamilton.

Telephone: (071) 81 433

Wanganui
PO Box 4322
Wanganui.

Telephone: (064) 37 612

Wellington
PO Box 55107
Waitangirua, Porirua.

Telephone: (04) 359 228

Whakatane
PO Box 370,
Whakatane.

Telephone: (076) 84 438

Whangarei
PO Box 712,
Whangarei.

Telephone: (089) 485 489

Index